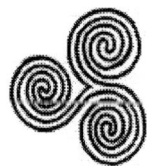

"No-one Knows What I'm Going Through"

The Secret Plague of Asbestos

The true story of Ellen Whitelaw who died of pleural mesothelioma, a vicious disease caused by exposure to asbestos. This book was written by her daughter who nursed her throughout her illness and ultimate death.

Asbestos causes many diseases in the human body including asbestosis, mesothelioma, chronic obstruction of the airways, emphysema, lung cancer and other cancers. The mesothelioma tumour can lie dormant in the human body for decades. But once it starts to grow sufferers have only weeks or months to live.

Included in this book are the stories of victims and their families; Steve McQueen the movie star, the blue asbestos mine & town of Wittenoom (Australia's worst disaster) with memories from the famous entertainer Rolf Harris, stories from Armley, Leeds, Hebden Bridge, Hull and Glasgow in the UK and the current situation in India where the use of asbestos is rising at the cost of workers who need jobs and who have not been told of the dangers they face.

British Library Cataloguing-in-Publication Data.
A catalogue record for this book is available from the British Library.

ISBN   978-0-9553021-1-4   0-9553021-1-0

"No-one Knows
What I'm Going Through"

The Secret Plague of Asbestos

B McKessock

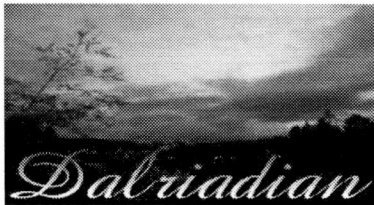

Contents

Introduction

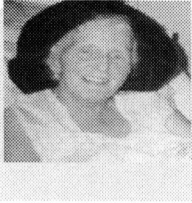

In 1995 I wrote a book about my mother, Ellen, and her suffering and ultimate death from Mesothelioma.

Mesothelioma The Story Of An Illness was taken from diaries I had written throughout my mum's illness and from pieces of information I managed to get together at that time.

I contacted several people by letter & telephone and visited some at home. People who were also suffering from asbestos related diseases. Every one of them had a life story to tell and every one of them went through the hell that asbestos causes to the human body. I still remember the stories I was told from every single person.

This is an update of that book. Looking back, I realise how raw everything was to me back then. With the passage of time, some of the wounds, frustration and anger which I felt back then have diminished. But the emotional scars are still there.

I hope this book reaches some people out there, even to let them know that they are not alone. And I hope I can do some justice to the stories and the friendships I made back 1993, the year of my mothers suffering and death.

Thank You To everyone who has ever talked, telephoned and written to me; my mum, Trudy McPhillips, Else Standen, Pat Standen, John McPherson, Nan McKenzie,

Nicholas McKenzie, Anne Grant, Irene Merrill, Dick Jackson, Iain McKechnie, Alan Dalton, Mr T Harkness, John Docherty, Bert Connor, Ben Hills, Rolf Harris, Clydeside Action On Asbestos, Hull Asbestos Action Group, The Asbestos Diseases Society of Australia and everyone who wished to remain anonymous.

I never got to properly thank Jimmy Willis, Martin Moffat, Harry McCluskey and Andrew Rae, the men who spoke up for my mum by giving details to our lawyers. Thank You.

BMcK July 2006

Asbestos

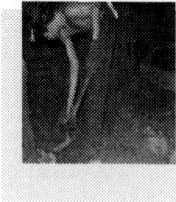

The Magic Mineral

Asbestos is a naturally occurring mineral found all over the world and has been mined on every continent and used by humans for centuries[1].

There are two groups; **chrysolite** and **amphibole**s.

Chrysolite (white) comes from serpentine rock. Its fibres are soft and curly.

Amphiboles has five distinct types; amosite (brown or grey), anthophyllite (white), crocidolite (blue), tremolite (white) and actinolite (white). Their fibres are small and straight.

The fibres of asbestos are so small that two million of them could fit onto a pinhead and they are invisible to the naked eye. Chrysolite (white asbestos) is the most abundant on Earth and has been found in large quantities in Canada. Crocidolite (blue asbestos) has only

---

[1] Photograph of a miner at Wittenoom, Asbestos Diseases Society of Australia

been found in South Africa and Australia. It has been proven to be at least sixty times more dangerous than white asbestos. However, traces of blue asbestos can be found amongst white and brown, making them just as dangerous to humans.

<u>All types of asbestos are known to cause cancer.</u>

The mineral was named 'asbestos' by the ancient Greeks who discovered it on Cyprus. It was incredibly resistant and could not be destroyed, so they called it 'inextinguishable' (asbestos).

There are bowls that are over 4,000 years old made of clay and asbestos which have been found in Finland.

History has given us clear warnings about asbestos. Over two thousand years ago Roman slaves were given facemasks when they wove asbestos fibres into cloth. Their masters realised the slaves became sick when working with the mineral.

In the 19th and 20th centuries asbestos was big business in the industrial world. By the end of the 1800's it was being mined and shipped across the world to be processed for widespread use. In Manchester and Birmingham factories sprung up where workers, mainly women, spun and weaved asbestos fibres. Health problems quickly appeared amongst them. Most of the women were in their 30's. They developed chesty coughs, they sickened, and then they died. The Lady Inspector of Factories wrote, in 1898, that workers amongst asbestos had more injuries (sickness) than any other workers she was aware of.

In 1906 the first death ever to be scientifically proven to have been caused by asbestos exposure brought to light the true killing nature of the mineral. A young man, age 33, was the last survivor of 10 men who had worked in a dust-covered room at an asbestos textile plant. The autopsy showed conclusively that he was killed by asbestos. It was another 20 years before the disease was named: asbestosis.

In 1930 a study was done on asbestosis. Merewether, a doctor from the Home Office, and Price, a ventilation engineer, examined 363 men and women who had been working with or in the vicinity of asbestos. Of the 363 people, 127 had asbestosis and Merewether & Price concluded that only 6 months exposure was enough to cause the disease. And that after 20 years exposure most of the workers would be expected to have the disease.

Even after reports such as there, nothing was done to protect workers in the UK or Europe from the effects of exposure to asbestos.

In 1939 World War II broke out. Asbestos related products were in demand for the war effort. The gas masks held out to the military and civilians contained asbestos in the breathing filter.

The twentieth century saw the mining of asbestos became very big business. Large international companies pulled it out of the ground and exported it all over the world, in its raw state and as products. It was hailed as 'the magic mineral' and it was used for almost everything.

After processing, raw asbestos loses its original colouring and all types and groups look the same to the naked eye. Only tests done in a laboratory can distinguish between them at this stage.

Resistant to heat and corrosion, asbestos fibres are strong and flexible and were used in;

> building & insulation materials, cement, pipes, fire resistant coatings on ships etc, structural girders, car brake linings, clutch plates, rubber, plastic, rope, boiler & pipe packing, pipe coverings, insulation blocks & boards, insulation jackets, spray-on structural heat insulation, electrical insulation tape, transformers, condensers, cables, conduits, electrical wire insulation,

spark plugs, switch boxes, circuit breakers, gaskets, bearing packing, seals, conveyor belting, wall sheets, gas pipes, water pipes, sewage pipes, reinforced asphalt, vinyl floor tiles, linoleum, panels, partitions, clapboard, asphalt siding & shingles, putties, ceiling boards, millboard, stucco, plaster, artificial wood, sound proofing, acoustic tile facings, paint, caulking, asbestos felt, cloth, sheets, blankets, curtains (including fire curtains in theatres), ribbon, artificial snow, filler in rubber goods, welding electrodes, cigarette filters, gas mask filters, filter cloths, filter pads, filter paper, catalyst supports for sulphuric acid production, water proof bearing & packing, cardboard, paper boat hulls, aeroplane wings, lamp wicks & burners, prison cell padding, fire hoses, mail bags, motion picture screens, frying pan handles, rocket re-entry nosecones, piano padding, military helmet lining, cartridges, car undercoating, fire proof safety clothing, life jackets, moulds, pottery & sculpture clay, ironing boards, pot holders, table pads, oven gloves and children's play dough, the filters of beer, fruit juice, whisky and medicines.

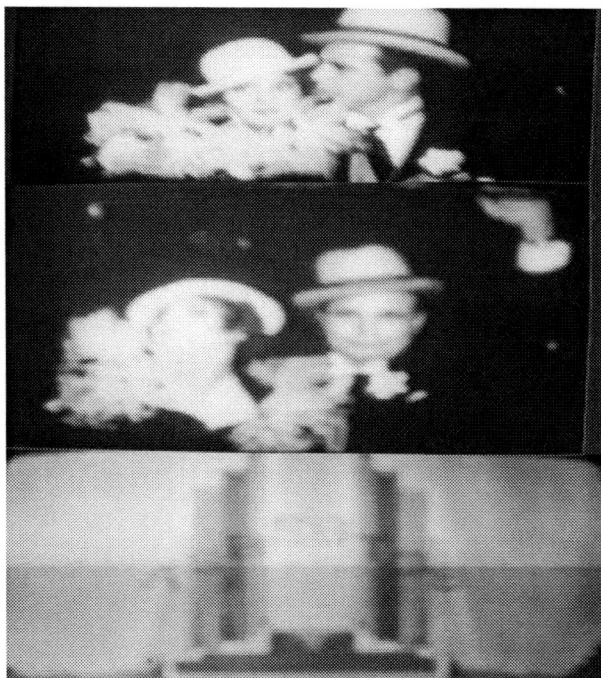

*From the film 42ⁿᵈ street, note the asbestos curtain
the male actor pulls down (1933)[2]*

Talcum powder was laced with it (wonderful for baby's bottom and think of all the women out there who use talc for personal hygiene) and children's sweets, remember those 'cigarette sweets'? Condoms, dusted with talc, have also been found to contain asbestos. In the early 1990's there were cases of genital and ovarian cancer amongst women in the UK, all caused by talcum powder that contained asbestos.

---

[2] Stills from 42ⁿᵈ Street (1933), Warner Bros. Studios

Asbestos is found in houses, schools, hospitals, shipyards, ships, roofs, floors, walls and many homes in the UK have an asbestos cement water tank in their attic.

Smoking is a major cause of cancer. Asbestos was used in the filter tips of cigarettes and in the paper that covered the tobacco.

Russia, the world's main producer of asbestos for several decades, produces more asbestos than any other country. The toxic waste, contamination and pollution that were hidden behind the iron curtain were revealed to the world when the Soviet Union fell. Conditions in the asbestos mines and factories were horrendous, and much worse than in the west.

When the threat asbestos posed to human health became abundantly clear in the 1960's it's use in the industrial world was diminished. The UK government banned blue asbestos in 1971.

Asbestosis is not the only disease cause by exposure to asbestos. It also causes lung cancer, cancer of the bowel, cancer of the stomach, cancer of the oesophagus, mesothelioma, pleural thickening, pleural plaques, emphysema, chronic bronchitis and chronic obstruction of the airways.

Diseases of Asbestos

Asbestosis

Asbestosis is a type of scarring or fibrosis of the lungs. Asbestos fibres that have been inhaled into the lungs cause it. Exposure to asbestos has usually occurred over several years and most people, mainly men, have worked closely with asbestos in shipyards or factories.

The latent period, the time it takes to develop asbestosis from the time of exposure, is 15 – 30 years.

One sufferer described asbestosis as feeling as if his lungs were slowly filling up with wet concrete. The lungs lose their elasticity making breathing increasingly difficult. Chest pains are common along with a rattly cough.

The lungs can become distorted, due to scarring in the lungs and scar tissue, and adhesions may develop in the lung, the diaphragm and in the outer lining of the heart.

There is no cure.

Cancers & Carcinomas

A carcinogen is any substance that produces cancer. Carcinoma of the larynx, abdomen (including the intestine, peritoneum, oesophagus and stomach), and bowel have all been linked to asbestos exposure.

Cancers of the ovary, hoemopoitic (blood forming) system, breast and mesothelioma in the lining of the testes have appeared.

Emphysema, Chronic Bronchitis & Chronic Obstruction of the Airways (COAD)

Emphysema is a disease that causes the destruction of the alveoli walls. Alveoli are small sacs in the lungs, which control the flow of air and blood. The partially destroyed lungs lose the power to work properly and the sufferer finds breathing difficult.

Chronic bronchitis is a disease where the sufferer's air passages become inflamed. It can be caused by smoking, by inhaling dust or pollution and by viral infections. Sufferers usually have a cough and mucus build up.

COAD (chronic obstruction of the airways) is a rather vague disease. It is similar to emphysema and chronic bronchitis. There is an obstruction in the airflow.

Normally associated and attributed to smoking, research ahs uncovered evidence that all of these diseases can be caused by exposure to dust and coal. In many cases, the sufferer has been a non-smoker and has never smoked.

These diseases are caused by exposure to dust. They **do not** 'run in the family' as is sometimes commonly, and mistakenly, believed.

Lung Cancer

Usually associated with cigarette smoking, lung cancer can also be caused by exposure to asbestos. The latency period is about 20 years and, if caught in time, a lung replacement has occasionally enabled a sufferer to recover.

Asbestos and smoking have a multiplicative effect on lung cancer development. Smokers amongst asbestos workers are 8 times more at risk of getting lung cancer than smokers who do not work with asbestos.

Mesothelioma

Probably the most horrific of all diseases caused by asbestos, is mesothelioma. It is a tumour, which grows inside the lining of the lung or inside the lining of the abdomen. It has also been known to grow inside the lining of the testes.

Pleural mesothelioma, inside the lining of the lung, causes the sufferer to experience increasing breathlessness and pains in the back or chest. As the tumour grows inside the lining, it stops the lung from functioning properly. If the lung cannot function, the sufferer cannot breath. *(see chapter 'Mesothelioma' for more information)*

The latency period is the longest and can be anything from 10 – 65 years. Once diagnosed the sufferer has only months to live.

There is no cure.

Pleural Thickening & Pleural Plaques

Asbestos fibres sometimes work their way out of the lung to the lining of the lung – the pleura. Pleural plaques can occur here and in the lining of the chest wall. Plaques usually develop before fibrosis although the plaques themselves do not become malignant.

Pleural thickening occurs when the asbestos fibres cause a thickening of a large pleural area. The sufferer becomes breathless as lung movement is restricted by the disease.

Plaques are similar to thickening but appear in small individual areas rather than one large one. Again, pain and breathing problems are usual.

There is no cure.

Mesothelioma

There are two main types of mesothelioma; **pleural** and **peritoneum.** Pleural mesothelioma occurs in the lining of the lungs and peritoneum mesothelioma, the rarer of the two, occurs in the lining of the abdomen.

Pleural Mesothelioma

Inside the chest are two lungs, which are protected by the rib cage. In between the ribs are muscles. These muscles, along with the diaphragm, are essential for breathing. The part of the brain, which controls breathing, receives signals from the body about how much oxygen is required to breathe. In turn, the brain sends messages along the nerves to these muscles. This allows the correct amount of air to be breathed in and out.

The lungs really are an incredible breathing machine. Inside each lung is a mass of fine tubes and the lung itself is like a sponge. The smallest of the fine tubes have ends that are called alveoli. These alveoli are tiny air sacs and there are about 300 million of them.

On the outside of the lung is the pleura, which is a lining tissue. It lies between the lung and the chest wall and it is wrapped around the lung. It has two membranes or layers and in between these two layers is the pleural cavity. Inside the pleural cavity is a small amount of fluid. As we breathe the two layers of the pleura slide back and forth over each other, allowing the lung to contract and expand.

Mesothelioma is a tumour, which grows inside the pleural cavity, hindering the sliding movement of the two layers and causing the lung to not function properly. The victim loses the capacity to breathe.

The first symptoms are breathlessness, chest pains and tiredness. The pleural cavity may start to fill up with fluid and a cough or a fever may develop.

As the tumour grows it fills the pleural cavity. Lung movement becomes restricted and eventually the tumour may fill most or the entire cavity. The victim cannot breathe properly and the heart must work harder to pump what oxygen there is in the body, around the body. Heart failure is not uncommon.

As the tumour grows the pleura thickens. A normal pleura has the thickness of a thin piece of paper but when mesothelioma takes hold, the tumour can grow to several inches in thickness and totally enclose the lung. Under this pressure the lung collapses.

Pleural tumours have been recorded for the last 200 years, but there has been some debate about whether or not they are the same, or different, from normal lung cancer. Only in the last 30 years have they been considered as a separate disease.

Peritoneum Mesothelioma

Peritoneum mesothelioma is very similar to pleural mesothelioma except it develops in the lining of the abdomen. It causes, over time, the victims stomach to swell. It is rarer than pleural mesothelioma.

* * * * * * *

Most cases of mesothelioma are caused by direct or indirect exposure to asbestos dust or fibres. Exposure to high levels of asbestos in a short period of time or exposure to low levels of asbestos over a long period of time can induce mesothelioma. Just one small instant of exposure could be enough. If the asbestos fibres lodge themselves in the victim's body, the chances of developing mesothelioma are relatively high. What triggers the disease is the amount of asbestos fibres, which are left in the lung or abdomen after exposure.

There is a long delay between exposure and obvious signs of the tumour, it can be anywhere from 10 to 65 years. In most cases the period appears to be 30 – 40 years.

Because of the rarity of mesothelioma (although increasing cases are coming to light as each decade passes), there is no cure. Chemotherapy, radiotherapy and surgery have been ineffective with only a small number of people gaining any short-term benefit.

Nerves around the lungs can become irritated and cause pain to the victim. Acupuncture and nerve block operations have been tried on patients, the idea to freeze or kill off irritated nerves in order to relieve some of the pain, homeopathy, aromatherapy and reflexology have also been attempted. However pain control, through drugs, is usually the only thing that can be done.

Once mesothelioma has been diagnosed the average time span of life left is about 7 months. The initial cause of the disease, those fibres in the body, may lie silent and dormant for decades. It is a time bomb. It is now widely believed that a biopsy will speed up the growth rate of the tumour. Without a biopsy some people have lived for 3 years.

Ignorance about mesothelioma and asbestos is rife. Those in the medical profession know, or say the know, very little about it. The general public know even less.

In 1992 someone we knew, after hearing he had mesothelioma, remarked

"It's not as bad as I thought. It's not cancer".

By 1993 he was dead.

The tumour that is mesothelioma resembles a horse's saddle. And it grows inside the human body.

"The actual tumour which mesothelioma produces is worse than any horror film could imagine", Iain McKechnie (Clydeside Action on Asbestos) said in 1994. "It is hideous. The tumour is thick and hard. It's as if it is made of really tough leather. It is hard and horny – extremely tough".

And a leading pathologist once said,

"Once you see mesothelioma you never forget it".

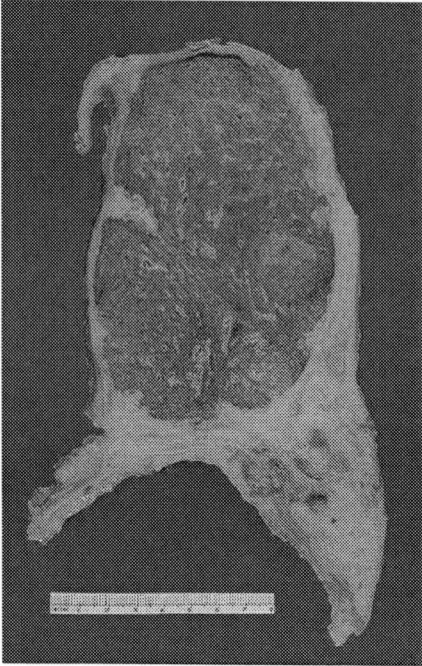

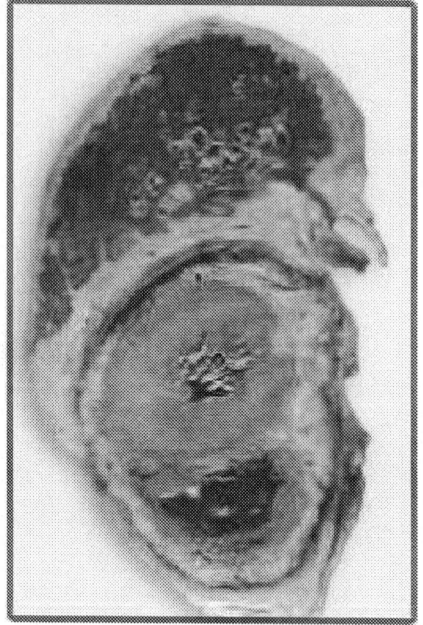

The Mesothelioma tumour (white)
inside the lung (dark area)[3]

[3] Photos (left) from Spencer S Eccles Health Sciences Library
http://medstat.med.utah.edu/WebPath/LUNGHTML/LUNG081.
html and (right) Asbestos Network
http://www.asbestosnetwork.com/health/he_meso.htm

Asbestos is the *only* known cause of mesothelioma. Or is it?

In the 1970's the small Turkish village of Karain had an outbreak of mesothelioma. The only problem was that there was no asbestos there. In 1978 a study discovered that volcanic activity had thrown out zeolites, volcanic silicates that have fibres very similar to asbestos fibres.

Replacements or alternatives have been used in the UK since the 1930's. Glass fibre was one of these and it also has fibres that are very similar to asbestos. In the 1960's 'glass fibre pneumoconiosis' (fibre glass lung scarring) was causing asthma, bronchitis, chest pain, breathing & nose problems, pneumonia, sore throats and coughs.

In 1976 an English family; mum, dad and 2 children, and their dog developed chest and breathing problems. The dog had to be put down. It was discovered that the dog had cancer in his lungs. Inside the dogs lungs were glass fibres. The family had recently installed a new central heating system and the air-duct lining was made of glass fibre.

Substitutes for asbestos, which mimic the length and width of asbestos itself, are a serious risk to human health.

Towns, Factories, Ships

Old Town, Hebden Bridge

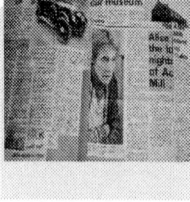

Cape Asbestos

The year is 1974 and the people of Wodsworth, otherwise known as Old Town Hebden Bridge, are concerned about the growing number of asbestos related deaths in the area.

Acre Mill, which stands at the top of the hill above the town, was once an asbestos factory and many people in this small Yorkshire town worked there. So far over 150 of them are dead or dying from asbestosis or mesothelioma. That number would rise in the future.

In production for over 30 years, the asbestos factory (owned by Cape Asbestos) was eventually closed in 1971. The people who worked there were never told of the dangers of asbestos and mothers & fathers took the deadly dust, stuck to their clothes, unknowingly home to their children.

Women ate their lunch amongst the fibres, even playing games with raw asbestos by making wigs and carrying on for a laugh.

Cape Asbestos Ltd (now Cape Industries) was the 2nd largest multinational asbestos company in the UK. At Acre Mill raw asbestos was made into asbestos textile products.

In all the time the factory was open the Factory Inspectorate never once prosecuted the owners even although conditions at the factory were found to be in violation of the British government's 1931 Asbestos Regulations. The Inspectorate, who should have been protecting the health of the workers & families never ensured that Cap handled asbestos in a safe way.

Brian Schnacke, an ex-employee, recalled how the extractors rarely worked because they were blocked and he and fellow workers often stood in blue dust up to a foot deep.

By 1974, Cape had paid out approx £400,000 to victims, no cases of which ever went to court. By 1979 the cost had risen to £2 million.

The mill was taken over by Raedaeln Ltd, a synthetic fibre processor and manufacturer. The Inspectorate insisted that the mill was clean (they cleaned it 3 times) and that there was absolutely no danger from asbestos.

In the next few years a Hebden Bridge Asbestos Group sprang up. Public meetings were called and the Old Town residents demanded to know what had been going on at Acre Mill. They wanted an inquiry.

More cases of asbestosis and mesothelioma appeared. By 1979 there had been 77 known cases of deaths; 57% lung cancer or mesothelioma, 24% heart failure, 14% pneumonia and 5% asbestosis.

Asbestos claimed the lives of 6 people in one family. A man who had worked at the mill for only 9 weeks at the age of 35, developed lung disease and died of mesothelioma when he was 48.

A government enquiry was set up and Cape spent £500,000 on an advertising campaign to convince people that asbestos was safe.

The townspeople were also concerned about where asbestos had been dumped. Where was it? Was it dangerous? In response Cape sent their own set of investigators to dumping grounds and assured the public that there was absolutely nothing to worry about. No asbestos, everything's fine, it's all perfectly safe.

Some asbestos, which had been found at Midgley and Carr Head, Pecket Well, the public were assured, no danger and was well covered up.

A theatrical play about the Hebden Bridge Massacre (as it was called) was performed in the town in August 1978 by a northern group. The play was based on one of the mill's ex-employees, Arthur Montgomery, who died of asbestosis the same month. The theatre group were subsequently sacked.

In 1980 part of the now half demolished Mill was transformed into a classic car museum. The Massacre was almost forgotten. By this time, however, 262 ex-mill workers out of a total of approx 2,200 people had an asbestos related disease. (Many ex-workers have never been traced because after the war, immigrants to the UK were employed there).

In 1982 ITV screened a television documentary Alice, A fight for life, which focused on Alice Jefferson, a woman fighting for her life against mesothelioma.

The tragedy of Acre Mill was once again in the spotlight. By now over 100 people were dead with another 300 diagnosed.

Plans were drawn up to have Acre Mill demolished and the site around it cleared. Suggestions of a car park for the museum and a children's play area were put forward and the local council were not amused when a member of the Asbestos Group claimed to have found asbestos (which was later analysed and found to be asbestos) in the area. The group were accused of hindering the clean up operation and the site was eventually landscaped and grassed over.

A member of staff at the Halifax Environmental Health office told me (in February 1994) that the site of the old mill was now a park. "Perfectly safe, it's all clean", he told me, although he became agitated at my questions.

When I went to the local post office at Wodsworth I wondered if people remembered the old mill or were even aware that it ever existed. The impression I had was that it was forgotten. How many children now played on the 'park'?

The Scout Road Tip was on of Cape's dumping grounds and, in 1993, the West Yorkshire Management Authority discovered asbestos on the surface of the soil. Public pathways had been closed off, animal burrowing and landslips had brought previously covered asbestos waste up to the surface.

By the end of the 1980's the asbestos related death toll in Old Town was over 200. That number would increase.

"I was 5 years old when I lost my mother to this terrible illness.

I am glad my mum didn't die in vain, I am glad she has not been totally forgotten.

That was the sole reason she made that program, to show the public what a dangerous substance asbestos is and to make the companies that used this stuff come out of the woodwork and take responsibility for the loss of life of many people in the local area.

I feel very strongly that we should keep this subject out in the open, so we never let anything like this happen again.

I think there should be some sort of a memorial at the site that was once Acre Mill for people to see and remember.

We cannot afford to stop remembering"[4]

Patsy Jefferson, daughter of Alice, who featured in the documentary *Alice, a Fight for Life*

29ᵗʰ April 2003

---

[4] Source : http://www.hebdenbridge.co.uk/features/acremill.html

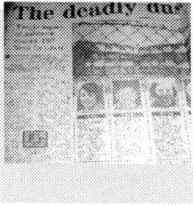

Armley, Leeds & Mumbai

JW Roberts, T&N, Hindustan

Armley & Leeds, UK

In 1993 the town of Armley near Leeds appeared on the pages of British newspapers. The reason? The town had an 'unusual' epidemic.

Mesothelioma had claimed the lives of at least 180 people in the town. An old asbestos factory, which had closed in 1958, had spread the lethal dust around the town exposing men, women and children.

The factory, JW Roberts, was taken over in 1921 by one of the largest asbestos producers in the world – Turner & Newall (now T&N). Asbestos snowdrifts were a common sight in the streets as the factory bellowed its poison from its chimneys. Inside the building workers were covered from head to toe in white dust. Outside, the kids played in it.

Children sitting on their fathers lap in the evening were exposed to the dust on his clothes. Women who washed those clothes were exposed. Outside homes, dust gathered on the windowsills and rooftops. Inside it became engrained in carpets and furnishings.

Residents of Armley recalled how factory employees came home with their coats and clothes covered in asbestos. Walking through their homes, they'd leave behind a trail of dust, fibres and 'fluff'.

Irene Merrill, a member of the local campaign for an asbestos-free Armley (c 1995) said "I've got asbestos in the door hinges and in the windows of my house. I don't clean in the crevices because I might disturb it". Asked why she still lived there she replied, "This is my home. I've got roots here and family".

When the campaign began against T&N many locals, particularly of the older generation were horrified that their town would be dragged into the media and get unwanted, bad publicity.

Irene said "At first some of the older folk were annoyed at us for kicking up a fuss about asbestos. They thought we were just causing trouble. But I think now they're beginning to realise that we're not just fighting for us, we're fighting for our kids. So now they support us just that little bit more".

T&N denied all responsibility saying that they were not aware that deaths in the town from mesothelioma were linked to their factory. Evidence, uncovered in 1993, proves that they lied.

Residents of the town couldn't sell their homes because of the asbestos. They became trapped in the mortgage money pit. As many homes, bought from the council and now owner-occupied, the local council wanted the residents to pick up the bill for decontamination. T&N, when asked by local campaigners to help, replied in a letter (c 1993)

> The Armley factory to which you refer was owned and operated by JW Roberts Limited. That company was, and still is, a wholly owned subsidiary of T&N plc. That fact alone does not give rise to any legal liability on this company's part.

JW Roberts Ltd began as a family business in 1870, set up by John William Roberts who died in 1896. The company produced low-pressure steam gland and water pumping packings and asbestos was introduced sometime before the 1900. John's wife and 3 sons; Clifford, Norman & John, continued the family business into the new century. When the company was amalgamated with Turner & Newall Ltd, Clifford Roberts joined the original board of directors of the 'new' company.

One of the uses of asbestos at the factory was as insulation for the boilers of steam locomotives. Sacks of crude asbestos would be laid over these massive boilers, which were several feet long and high, and there was often a lot of it spilt when the sacks were later removed.

By 1906 even the very sacks themselves were made of asbestos cloth[5]

Turner & Newall were attracted to JW Roberts because of the latter's close relationship with the Washington Chemical Company. Unlike other manufacturers who used white asbestos, Washington Chemical used raw blue asbestos, supplied by Roberts, in their Magnesia Plastic product.

JW Roberts were producing blue asbestos textiles, packings, jointings and insulation mattresses for locomotive boilers by 1918. In Kimberley, South Africa, were diamond mines and it was in this area that blue asbestos was found, mined and shipped to Yorkshire.

By 1927, Armley was also producing blue asbestos yarns, corrugated asbestos paper, and asbestos felts. In 1930 the asbestos spraying process was introduced and the Roberts factory supplied sprayed asbestos coating for insulation to the British or other navies, merchant ships, oil tankers and for buildings and railway carriages throughout the world.

---

[5] Remember, the first death scientifically proven to have been caused by asbestos was in 1906

So successful was the sale of Armley products that, in 1950, Turner & Newall – now called Turner Brothers Asbestos Co Ltd – built a new factory at Hindley Green. This factory was to produce mattresses, spray fibre and blue asbestos textiles.

In 1958 the Armley factory was closed. The new owners were TAC Construction Materials Ltd of Manchester, a large firm that had links to asbestos and other materials.

Under a new name Turner & Newall opened a factory in Mumbai (Bombay) in India. It is still there and is still operating (*see following article on Mumbai*).

Half a tonne of blue asbestos was discovered in 4 Armley factories in February 1978. TAC (formerly TAC Construction Materials Ltd) spent approx £12,000 decontaminating the sites which they said they did from a moral – not legal – obligation.

Fifteen years later concrete, which had been poured over dumped asbestos at the back on one of the factories, began to crack and blue asbestos fibres were found inside. It was claimed that the original clean up operation was nothing more than a public relations exercise.

In the 1980's a spate of asbestos related deaths drew the attention of the local media particularly as some of the victims had not actually worked in the factories.

One victim, Margaret Ibbetson, had worked in a local co-op, which was near the Armley factory. She had never been in direct contact with asbestos but died at the age of 60 from mesothelioma.

Another victim, a 64-year-old woman, told how the local school was 100 yards away from the factory. She described how asbestos had covered the playground and children skipped and played in it. Agnes Whelan, who died aged 77 of mesothelioma, lived half a mile away from the factory.

The end of the 1980's brought to the public's attention more deaths caused by exposure to asbestos. Armley was a contaminated town and, even 30 years after the Roberts factory had closed, the death toll was still rising. And it would continue to do so.

As an Armley Asbestos Campaign group demanded an inquiry, Leeds City Council claimed to have known nothing about the town's contamination until 1988. Strangely, documents from the 1970's had mysteriously disappeared.

In 1993 Chase Manhattan, a multinational company began proceedings to sue T&N for the asbestos contamination of their New York office skyscraper. Unlike British lawyers, who were denied access to T&N's documents, Chase seized millions of papers from an English warehouse and shipped them back to the USA.

A memo, written by a T&N public relations officer, stated

> "I hope very much that we are never called upon to discuss Armley in the public arena"

Another internal, strictly confidential, memo reads

> "Public access to the information that we have could explode a bomb that would wreck T&N"

Mumbai, India

As asbestos became a dirty word in the Western world, the multinational corporations closed their factories and moved them east, into Africa, India and other parts of Asia.

In 1949 Asbestos Magnesia and Friction Material (AM&FM), formally Turner & Newall, opened a new factory in Sewri, Mumbai in India. This was moved to a new site in 1956 at Ghatkopar, Mumbai with a new name of Hindustan Ferodo. In 1990 the name changed to Hindustan Composites.

In 2005, V Murlidhar and Vijay Kanhere produced a study of asbestos related diseases at the factory. The study, *Asbestosis in an asbestos composite mill at Mumbai: A prevalence study* [6], was conducted by the Occupational Health & Safety Centre and the Worker's Union.

Permission to conduct the study within the factory was refused by Hindustan Composites and they also would not co-operate in the survey which was then conducted out-with the factory premises. Between 10th to 13th November 2004,

---

[6] Asbestosis in an asbestos composite mill at Mumbai: A prevalence study by V Murlidhar & Vijay Kanhere can be found here
http://www.pubmedcentral.nih.gov/picrender.fcgi?artid=1289287&blobtype=pdf

employees were approached at the factory gates and of the 232 permanent staff, 181 took part in the survey. The contract staff however, were apprehensive and did not take part. [7]

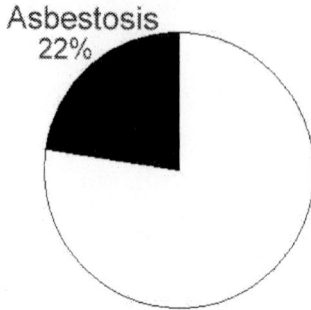

Asbestosis
22%

Percentage of the 181 employees studied who had asbestosis (in black)

Of the 181 workers studied, 41 (22%) had asbestosis and of these, over 80% of them worked in areas with high dust exposure.

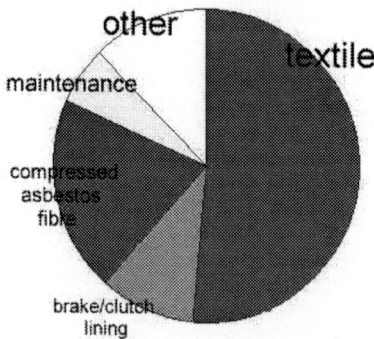

other
textile
maintenance
compressed
asbestos
fibre
brake/clutch
lining

Departments where the 41 employees with asbestosis worked *(see numbers & percentages below)*

---

[7] In 2003 Hindustan Composites forced a lock out which lasted for over 7 months. In 2004 production re-started with a reduced work force and with 110 people resigning 'voluntarily'

Dept	Textile	BCL	CAF	Maint	Other	**Total**
#	21	7	6	3	4	**41**
%	51%	17%	15%	7%	10%	**100 %**

Table 1 - Numbers of employees & percentages against department (of the 41 employees with asbestosis) {numbers have been rounded}

The departments with the highest dust exposure were Textile, BCL (brake & clutch lining) & CAF (compressed asbestos fibre) which was a total of 34 people (or 83% of the 41).

The study also found that employees were working with raw white asbestos, which entered the factory in bags and that they had no control or decisions over their working practices. Raw asbestos was then made into products such as textiles, cloth, rope, brake & clutch lining, compressed asbestos fibre and asbestos sheets.

The employees had also never been given any information from Hindustan Composites about the effects of asbestos and any other hazardous materials within the factory.

Since a total of 181 of a possible total of 232 current employees took part in the survey, this means that 22% (over a fifth) of the current employees were not examined so there is no way of telling how many of those people have asbestosis or an asbestos related disease.

It is also highly likely that employees who left the factory before 2004 were undiagnosed and may now be suffering or have died from asbestosis. If the sick leave or are forced to leave the *Healthy Worker Effect* takes place (i.e. those left are younger and healthier than those older employees who have been exposed for years), which gives a bias on the numbers and percentages in the results of any of study.

Without employees and their families knowing the facts about asbestos and with a lack of training for doctors in diagnosing these diseases (as well as deliberate non diagnosis and a social/cultural bias between management, professional and working people), across India, by 2005, of an estimated **100,000** workers who have been exposed to asbestos, **less than 30** have received any compensation.

The study concluded that
- ❖ all affected asbestos workers, including those who have been forced to leave employment, in India be medically certified and compensated

- ❖ there should be better control of asbestos use in India

❖ management should provide all information about the work process and its hazards, conduct medical check ups as mandated by law and give the medical records to the workers [8]

As in Armley and Leeds, those who work in and around asbestos factories take the dust home to their husbands, wives, children and other extended family. Indian culture would also include very extended families, living socially & closely together. The factories themselves pollute the area around them.

Therefore the affects and the eventual toll of asbestos will be much higher than any employee number.

And that toll will go on for decades to come.

---

[8] Ref Source for Mumbai, India Information & Data - Asbestosis in an asbestos composite mill at Mumbai: A prevalence study by V Murlidhar & Vijay Kanhere

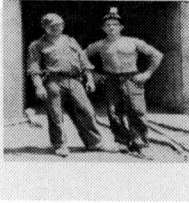

Wittenoom

Hancock, CSR, ABA

One of the most popular characters on British television today is a bearded Australian who sings songs about kangaroos, a three legged bloke and a song about two little boys. He is an entertainer, a singer, an artist and a player of strange musical instruments and cardboard! The words didgeridoo, wobble board, lagerphone and stylophone bring him to mind. Rolf Harris.

But he wasn't always an entertainer.. In 1948, as a young man, we worked for the summer in a mine. A blue asbestos mine. Wittenoom.

The town of Wittenoom is in the north west of Australia, about 1,600km north of Perth beyond the Great Sandy Desert.

It's a hot, dry, desolate place. And rough. When they weren't working in the mine the men drank, gambled, fought, gambled some more, fought some more and drank some more.

"It was the law of the jungle", remembered Rolf. "They were a real bunch of desperados, fighting all the time. They had no mercy".

Rolf had gone there for summer holiday work, on a break from university. He thought he could earn some money and do some painting, except the paint dried as soon as it hit the canvas.

"It must have been 120 degrees.. you had to drink water all the time, eat salt tablets. The men slept naked in tents, that's how hot it was", he said.

The mineshafts where most of the men worked, were only 3 feet high and miners would be bent double throughout their shifts. Rolf said, "the first time I walked into the mine, I crashed into the roof and knocked myself out. You were working in these tunnels so low you couldn't straighten up. There was dust everywhere.. around the shed where they crushed the asbestos, it was like a grey-blue haze.. It was murder".

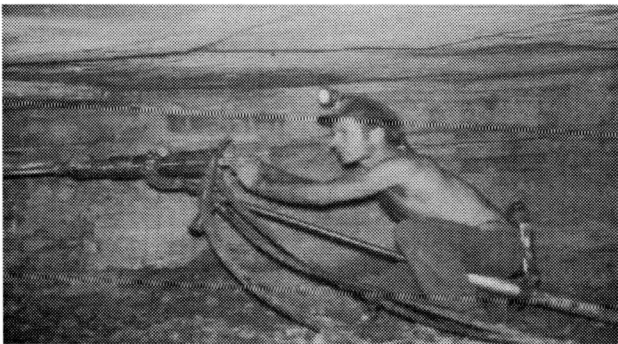

inside a mine at Wittenoom

Luckily he didn't have to work there for any longer than 3 months and was lucky to get out of mining altogether. "Eventually the man I was shovelling the rock with said he wouldn't work with me any more because I wasn't pulling my weight. Thank God for that. I was transferred to laying water pipes".

Yampire Gorge, near the small town of Wittenoom, was the blue asbestos seam, which was opened as a mine by Lang Hancock in the late 1930's. By 1940 the mine had produced 365 tonnes of blue asbestos, which was sold to an English asbestos company. The Colonial Sugar refining Company (CSR) joined forces with Hancock and a new company Australian Blue Asbestos (ABA) was set up to run the mine. The John Manville Corporation of America became their biggest customer.

Wittenoom became a boomtown and workers were recruited from all over the world. At the end of World War II, immigrants flocked to Australia for a better life. Many of these, mainly young men, ended up at Wittenoom; hundreds of Italians, Spaniards, Germans, Dutch, Yugoslavians, Poles, Hungarians & Greeks.

Up to 500 men worked at the mine at any given time but, because of the appalling conditions, the turn over was over 8,000, many of whom had been told by ABA how good the conditions

were and how nice the climate was. There was a
500% turnover of workers in some years
because most people wanted away from the
place as soon as they got there.

Working conditions were primitive, men tore
asbestos out by hand, trampled into jute sacks
by hands & feet and transported to ports by
horse & carts.

In the mill where raw asbestos was grounded
down to fibres, one worker remembered how
100-watt bulbs looked like candles and you
had to be up close to someone before you
could recognise him. The mill eventually got
an extractor, which didn't work. It blew dust
outside into the air covering offices and lawns.

The mine itself was hot, dusky and dark and,
until the 1960's, had no airshafts. Men crawled
on their knees, faces were caked in dust, in the
food shack men ate their meals off tables
covered in blue asbestos dust and used stringy
blue asbestos fibres as dental floss.

The men at Wittenoom were never warned of
the dangers of asbestos, in fact they played
with it, even using an air hose to blast it into
each other's faces as a joke.

Professor Eric Saint, a 29-year-old medical
graduate from Durham University was

horrified at what he saw in the summer of 1948. "It was horrendous, absolutely horrendous. There were no amenities, people were still living in tents and shacks. There were fights and mayhem going on everywhere".

Dr Saint[9] reported the barbaric medical facilities to the Public Health Department in Perth; wounds going septic because of filthy dressings, a filthy orderly, dust hanging like a cloud over the entire area, early examinations of young men with chest diseases, warnings of the dangers of asbestos, he repeatedly wrote damming reports. In one of his early reports he wrote

"ABA will produce the richest and most lethal crop of asbestosis in the world".

ABA, however, did nothing to make conditions cleaner or safer but chose instead to cover up the real facts about asbestos then later deny all responsibility for the deaths of their workers.

---

[9] Dr Saint went on to become one of the most highly respected and distinguished professors in Australia. He died in 1989.

The trade unions and health departments did nothing.

Vermiglio is a small village in the Italian Alps and in the 1950's nine young men set off to Australia for a great adventure. They arrived at Wittenoom. Arriving at the mine by aeroplane, the pilots main navigational aid was a blue-grey asbestos plume which shoot into the air. They were shocked and one later commented "we thought we were in Hell".

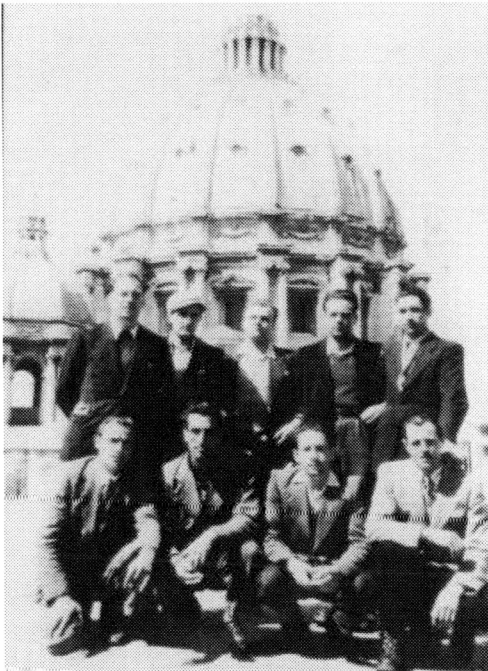

The Italians

Over 1,000 Italians passed through Wittenoom and years later, after returning home, all over Italy ex-Wittenoom miners began to sicken and die.

By 1989 five of those nine were dead or dying of an asbestos disease, one had been blinded by an explosion at the mine and in the Italian village of Abruzzi, 21 'Wittenoom boys' became ill.

Gino Casale, one of 4 brothers who'd been to the mine became concerned when 2 of his brothers became ill. "Something is going on", he said, "all the boys of Wittenoom are dying".

But it wasn't just the boys.

In 1979 Joan Joosten was dying of mesothelioma. She had worked at Wittenoom in the 1950's as a secretary. She sued ABA and lost. They claimed that when she worked for them mesothelioma was an unknown disease in the medical profession, so they were not to blame. Her appeal was set for the 10th March 1980, she died half an hour before it began.

The actual town of Wittenoom was 14 kilometres away from the mine. It was a normal, small town. Tailings (crushed rock) were supplied free to anyone who wanted them so they were carted around by truck and used in roads, the airport, the school and in the driveways of houses. In all over 30,000 tonnes were used in the town.

Great pillars of dust would spring up in the town – they called them willy-willie's – sometimes right over family homes.

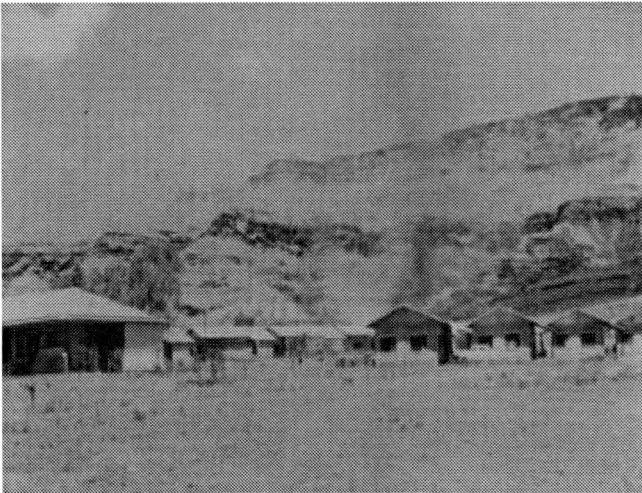

The town of Wittenoom, the dust cloud over the houses is raw blue Asbestos

Children played in the dust, men came home from the mine covered in it, the everyday fabric of home life was riddled with blue asbestos. Asbestosis and mesothelioma killed mothers, fathers and children.

The mine was closed in 1966, with the first case of asbestosis in 1946 and first mesothelioma in 1961. CSR/ABA were sued for the first time in 1977 but the victim died before getting to court. By 1989 the known death toll was over 600 and across Australia the publicity surrounding the mine drove people, some only in their 30's, to their doctors. "I grew up in Wittenoom", they would say.

The mine is now abandoned. A sign bearing a skull and crossbones marks the spot. When the wind blows in a certain way blue tailings are carried down the gorge to the town where tourists can buy blue-black souvenirs to take home. There are no warnings, no danger signs, just souvenirs.

It is estimated that thousands of people will die because of exposure at Wittenoom, in Vermiglio the locals have renamed their cemetery 'Wittenoom'.

As recently as 1974 blue asbestos was still being used in Australia and by a cruel twist of fate Rolf Harris lost his father to asbestosis. He had worked in a power station. Rolf said,

> "My dad died of asbestosis in 1980 due, they think, to a period about 40 years earlier when the large turbine

broke down in the electricity power
station where he worked. For about a
month they had the stand-by turbine
going while they repaired the big one
and the alternative one ran very
ragged, shaking the whole place day
and night.

All the best water pipes were lagged
with asbestos cloth and dad said going
to work was like walking into a thick
grey fog every day. Later in 1979, he
got a bad persistent cough and was
very short of breath".

Wittenoom asbestos found it's way into docks
around the world. It was used in power
station, trains and gas masks made in England
in the 1940's. Think of all the people
unknowingly exposed, thousands and
thousands of people.

Val Doyle, a 49-year-old wife and mother was
the 6th member of her family to die, in 1989,
because of Wittenoom.

"They have committed genocide on my
family", she said.

Wittenoom has been called Australia's industrial Belsen [10]

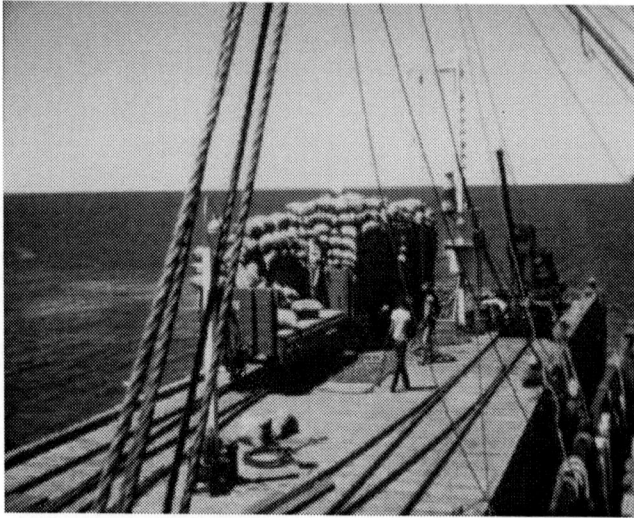

Wittenoom Asbestos being loaded to be shipped across the world

---

[10] Wittenoom information taken from Blue Murder by Ben Hills (Sun Books, Australia 1989) & Wittenoom – the worst disaster (Asbestos Diseases Society of Australia)
Photographs by Asbestos Diseases Society of Australia

Ships & Industry

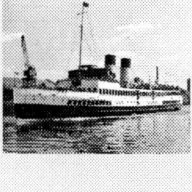

The shipyards along the river Clyde, from Dumbarton to Glasgow in Scotland produced some of the biggest and most magnificent ships in the world.

The cruise ship the *Queen Mary II* was built in 1933 and carried up to 1,500 passengers. Her last voyage was in 1978 and, in 1980, she was bought by a retail group and is now a floating pub, restaurant and nightclub at the Victoria Embankment in London.

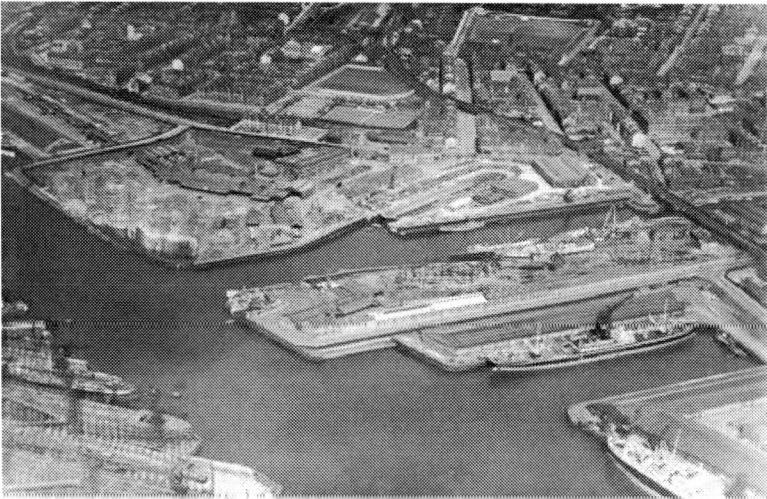

Clyde Shipyards 1930's

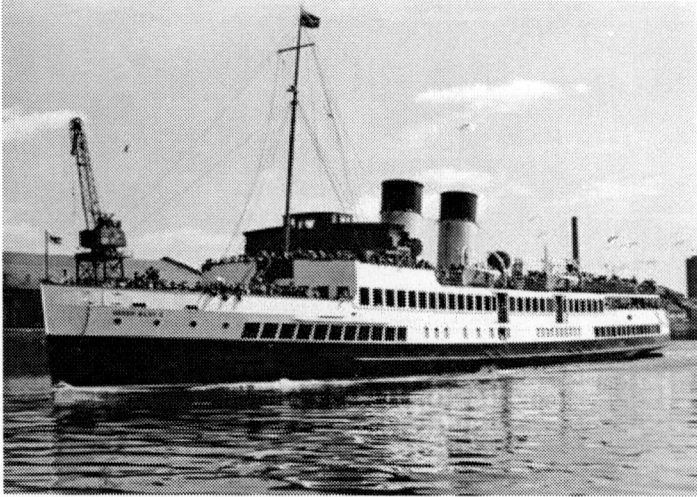

Queen Mary II 1955

These ships were built at a cost to the men and their families who worked in the shipyards. As the 20th century drew to a close, many of them had died or were dying of asbestos related diseases [11]

In Glasgow the Govan shipyards employed thousands of men. Young men left school at 14 and joined their fathers, uncles or cousins and in those days, until the 1970's when the shipyards began to close, a job was for life.

---

[11] Information from http://www.theglasgowstory.com
Photographs; Clyde Shipyards 1930' by Glasgow University Archive Services & Queen Mary II by Partick Camera Club (Glasgow Museums Collection)

Through-out the decades of the 1930's to the 1970's sacks of raw asbestos arrived at these docks. Dockers unloaded them and sat on them as they ate their lunch.

Where now Glasgow has pleasing blocks of upmarket flats and homes, there was once docks, an asbestos factory and dumping grounds. On the site of the old asbestos factory is a £180 million private hospital.

John MacPherson worked in the Clyde shipyards, "Monkey dung", he said, "It had asbestos in it. We used to mix it up and caked pipes with it for insulation"

There was asbestos 'snow' around the docks of Hull, Liverpool, Portsmouth and Belfast, in fact every major port in the UK. Tens of thousands of men worked at these docks as engineers, laggers, dockers, pipe fitters and more. And those men went home at night to family.

"He took it home to his marital bed", one sufferer told me as tales of wives dying of cervical cancer became common. "It killed his wife".

Dick Jackson was a lagger in Hull and first came into contact with asbestos in 1947. "I live with my fingers crossed", he told me. He became active in the campaign to have asbestos banned in 1970 and was committed to helping others.

He travelled the world attending conferences and lobbying. In 1992 Dick and the Hull Asbestos Action Group delivered a petition to the British government asking them to follow the policy of Scandinavia who had already banned asbestos.

In 1994 Dick was diagnosed with mesothelioma. He died on the 30th October the same year.

> *Dick, founder of the Hull Asbestos Action Group and stalwart anti-asbestos campaigner, began his working life as a thermal insulation engineer and was first exposed to asbestos when lagging pipes in the Hull dockyards. Exposure to asbestos continued throughout his working life and Dick died from mesothelioma only six weeks after the disease was diagnosed.*
>
> *Dick was a pivotal force in the British anti-asbestos movement for more than twenty years. During this time, he worked tirelessly on both a national and international level: assisting British victims in their struggle for compensation and liaising with a network of like-minded individuals and groups throughout Europe. Dick's enthusiasm, determination and humanity will be sorely missed.*

(British Asbestos Newsletter)

Naval warships, submarines, great ocean liners, the royal yacht, magnificent ships built in the UK were riddled with asbestos. No employee was ever told that asbestos was dangerous.

> "They never told us", one said, "They never said a word, not a fucking word that this stuff could kill you. Now I know. I bloody well know and it's too fucking late!"

All over the world asbestos companies have continually suppressed information, reports and documents which link asbestos to cancer.

Used mainly for insulation purposes, processed asbestos was used for many years in the shipbuilding and industrial sectors exposing many people, mostly men, to unknown health problems in their later years. Since the 1970's cases of mesothelioma have dramatically increased as people who were exposed to asbestos during the 1940's – 1970's, develop the disease.

Areas in the UK with a higher risk of mesothelioma are as follows;

Ship Building areas;

Scotland; West Dunbartonshire, East Dunbartonshire, Fife, Glasgow City, Inverclyde and Renfrewshire

England; Hartlepool, Middlesbrough, Redcar and Cleveland, Stockton-on-Tees, Tyne & Wear Metropolitan County, Blythe Valley, Barrow-in-Furness, Wirral, Isle of White, Medway, Portsmouth, Southampton, Fareham, Gosport, Havant, New Forest in Hampshire, Plymouth, Caradon in Cornwall and the Isle of Scilly.

<u>Railway Engineering areas;</u>

England; Crewe & Nantwich, Doncaster, Leeds, Derby, Eastleigh, Swindon

<u>Factories with raw asbestos areas;</u>

Sunderland in Tyne & Wear, Leeds, Calderdale, Thurrock, Castle Point in Essex, London, Dartford and Gravesham.

Deaths of females are 6 times lower than that of males. However, one significant point from the report mentions areas with significantly elevated female deaths which include those areas associated with the manufacture of gas masks during the war; Blackburn with Darwen, Chorley, South Ribble, Nottingham and Broxtowe in Nottinghamshire.

True Lives

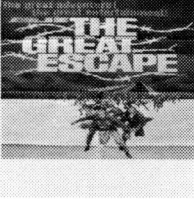

Steve McQueen
International Film Star

The great escape is one of Steve McQueen's best known and most successful films. Clydeside Action of Glasgow have a poster from that film on their wall. It shows Steve on a motorcycle. Scrawled across it are the words *no escape from asbestos.*

Steve McQueen was born on the 24th march 1930 in Indiana, USA. He never knew the father who walked out on him when he was a few months old. His teenage mother, who craved fun and excitement, regularly left him with other relatives while she went off to the bright lights and dancing.

Practically raised by his grandmother and his womanising uncle, he had an unstable childhood who grew up to be a moody, rebellious teenage, who then grew up to be a mysterious stubborn moody man.

After spending some time at Boys Republic, an institution for wayward boys, Steve joined the Merchant Marines, where he later jumped ship. He had and lost several dead-end and uneventful jobs. Always looking for a scam, he would steal in order to survive, or just to prove that he was smarter than the next guy. He often said if he hadn't been an actor, he would have been a criminal.

At the age of 21, he joined the New York City Neighbourhood Playhouse and his acting career began. He began by doing bit parts on stage and in 1956 appeared in his first film, *Somebody Up There Likes Me*. He was paid $19 a day and the star of the film was Paul Newman.

Over the next couple of years he made more appearances on television, stage and film but it was the successful 1958 TV series *Wanted: Dead or Alive* which caught the publics imagination and catapulted him to stardom.

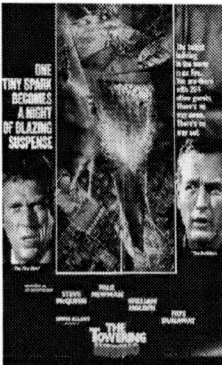

More film offers came in and his name began to creep up the credits to top billing. His percentage share of the 1974 film *The Towering Inferno* (which also starred his long time rival Paul Newman) and his salary grossed Steve over $12 million.

By the end of the 1970's Steve McQueen was the highest paid actor in the world.

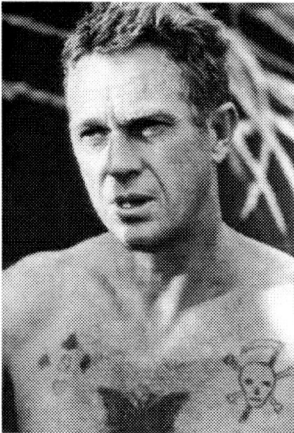

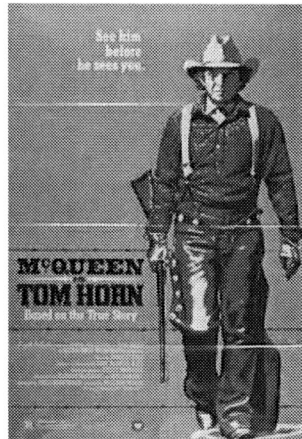

Papillion & Tom Horn

In 1978 he caught pneumonia and was unusually ill for a long time. It didn't seem to shake off and he developed a cough. He caught colds frequently afterwards. In January 1979 shooting began for a new film, the cowboy western *Tom Horn*. Steve was still feeling under the weather.

During the weeks of filming he became tired and breathless but he never let anyone on the set know. The wife of the first assistant director of the film, Cliff Coleman, was a nurse. Steve bombarded her with questions about lung diseases, what was pleurisy like?

Doctors could find nothing wrong with him and they decided that he had fungus on his lungs. The cause was probably damp sea air, they said. So, in response to his doctor's advice, he left his beach house for a ranch in the drier conditions of Idaho.

In the summer he had a lung biopsy and in September he began working on what would be his last film *The Hunter*. The first scenes to be filmed were stunts on top of a subway train. Steve refused to stand aside and let a stuntman do them and, even though he was ill, insisted on doing them himself.

Watching *The Hunter* one night you quickly became aware of how old Steve McQueen looked. He was only 49 years old but looked over 60. In one scene he chases a teenager over a roof. His body is not agile and you get the feeling he is in pain. His back was slightly hunched and many of his movements are stilted.

Robert Relyea, an old friend of Steve's, saw *The Hunter* in California when it opened in 1980. He hadn't seen Steve for a couple of years and he was shocked at the image he saw projected on the big screen. Robert was alarmed and deeply distressed at the way Steve moved. Clearly there was something very wrong and Robert realised that Steve was trying to cover his pain.

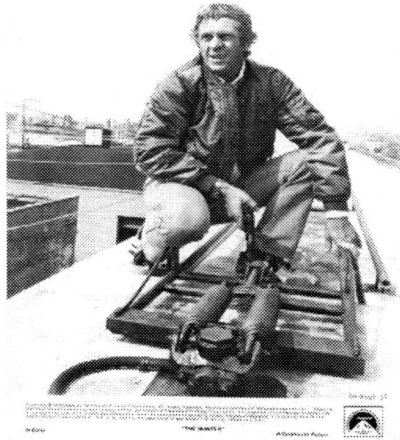

The Hunter

Steve developed an uncontrollable cough and became more and more breathless.

In December 1979 he checked in to a Los Angeles medical centre for tests. The results confirmed that he had **Peritoneum Mesothelioma.** He told his daughter Terry not to worry, as it wasn't a terminal disease. He didn't have cancer.

"I'm going to make it", he said.

Steve had always had a passion for cars, he was an excellent driver and he loved to race against the pros. Asbestos is found on the brake linings of cars and in the helmets & equipment used by drivers. He would also have been exposed to asbestos in some of his early jobs when he worked at construction sites and when he was in the armed forces.

In 1947, a 17 year old Steve McQueen joined the Marine Corps and spent some time in the Aleutian Islands. On one occasion, as the facility was being inspected by a general, he made himself a snack and heated a can of beans on top of a tractor engine. The can exploded and the contents went everywhere. His punishment was to spend 6 weeks in the brig where he was assigned to work in the hold of a ship.

The engine room, which he had to clean, had pipes covered in asbestos linings. The men were in the process of ripping out these linings and replacing them. The air was so thick with asbestos dust that the men could barely breath.

The ships of the US navy were riddled with asbestos, as were those of the British. Even the Queen's ship, the Royal Yacht Britannia had its asbestos removed in the 1960's. In 1994 an ex-member of the Queen's staff who had worked aboard the yacht died of an asbestos related disease. All ex-staff were immediately recalled for medical tests.

Over the next few months Steve tried every treatment he could including chemotherapy, radiation treatments and interferon, a new expensive anticancer drug. Nothing worked.

Only his very close family were told what was wrong with him. His first marriage, to Neile Adams, had lasted 16 years and the couple had 2 children Terry and Chad.

The film actress Ali McGraw, his co-star in the 1972 film *The Getaway* became his second wife in 1973. They divorced in 1977.

His third wife was Barbara Minty, a successful model. They had been dating for several months before he became ill. They married on the 16th January 1980. It was a very low-key and casual affair. Some of Steve's friends resented Barbara as they saw her as a newcomer. But it was she who, over the next few months, tried to help Steve battle his illness to the bitter end.

Together his family conspired to keep the press at bay as rumours raged around Hollywood. *Steve McQueen has cancer. He is dying.* Steve denied it all. Neile and Ali lunched with journalists and talked about the virus Steve was beating. An American magazine published an article about the hopelessness and doom of McQueen's situation. Threatening to sue, Steve's' response was that he didn't have terminal cancer, he had terminal fury.

Desperate to find a cure he tried unorthodox treatments. He tried a non toxic cure for cancer (or the so-called Washington doctor who discovered it claimed) of nutritional therapy, a diet of organic fruits, juices and vitamins. It didn't work.

He started telephoning and visiting old friends and still refused to believe that he was dying. If someone asked if he had cancer or was dying he would answer that it was all lies and he was fine.

In reality his body was rapidly deteriorating. He was losing weight, his cheeks sunk, his coughing got worse and he had more trouble breathing.

Barbara nursed him as he attended San Fernando Medical Centre for chemotherapy. They lived in a motor home behind the hospital because Steve would have been recognised if he had gone in as a normal patient. He didn't want the press to know what was going on.

When *The Hunter* was released in July 1980 critics slammed Steve's performance. "Tired Daredevil" was how one put it. What they didn't know was that they were watching a dying man.

Three days after the premier Steve and Barbara drove to Mexico and Steve entered the Plaza Santa Maria Clinic in Tijuana, a clinic run by the same doctor who had given him the nutritional diet. The treatment was very unorthodox but he was desperately trying to cling to life and time was running out.

The doctor, Dr Kelly was actually a dentist. He had been suspended from practising dentistry and had been cited in Texas for practising medicine without a license. He moved to Mexico.

Steve was subjected to special diets, coffee enemas, vitamins; cattle cell injections, shampoos, massages, psychotherapy and prayer. He did not use painkillers but relied on prayer. He told his friend Elmar Valentine that he would take the pain, every bit of it – even if it killed him.

He developed allergies and would lie awake night after night in utter agony. He would rant and rave, complain and throw things at Barbara. He would cry. The only people he allowed near him were Barbara, Neile, Terry and Chad. He refused Ali's requests to see him.

Neile sadly told friends that it would be better for them to remember him as he was, as they wouldn't recognise him now.

She tried to get him back to the USA and into a proper hospital. He refused. An old friend, Don Gordon, even proposed kidnapping him using a helicopter and guns!

In the meantime the press descended on the clinic. The going rate for a photograph of Steve McQueen was $50,000.

As his condition deteriorated he decided he'd like to spend Christmas with his family all together. Then, realising he would never see another Christmas, he told Neile to forget the whole thing.

"I won't be here", he said.

After all of the denials, on the 2nd October 1980 Steve issued a joint statement with his doctors. It stated that he had cancer but that he was responding to treatment.

Steve said, "I say to all my fans and friends, keep your fingers crossed and keep the good thoughts coming. All my love and God bless you".

Through this apparent recovery the clinic received a lot of media attention. Dr Kelly insisted that some of Steve's tumours had disappeared, that new ones were not appearing and that those which were left were becoming light *"like cotton candy"* [12]

---

[12] See the earlier chapter Mesothelioma (p16) for what actually happens in the human body re. this tumour

On the 24th October Steve and Barbara drove home to their ranch in Santa Paula . His daughter Terry visited him there.

"He wasn't afraid of dying", she said. She was deeply saddened at the amount of pain he was in but was proud of how he fought it. "He fought it up to the very end".

In the meantime Barbara continued to nurse, put up with his fits of anger and depression and, in response to a friend saying it must be tough for her, sadly answered "you wouldn't believe it".

He grew weaker, he couldn't breath. For the very first time he started to take morphine to ease his agony. The tumour in his abdomen had caused his stomach to swell up.

The doctors at the clinic in Mexico wanted to operate on this abdominal 'dead tumour' as they said it was putting pressure on his internal organs. American doctors warned that his heart would not withstand surgery. However Steve decided to return to Mexico to have the operation.

On 6th November, at the Clinica de Santa Rosa in Juarez, Steve McQueen underwent major surgery. A five pound tumour was removed from his abdomen, another was attached to his liver, his entire intestine was covered in cancerous cells and his right lung was cancerous.

He survived. He opened his eyes, gave the thumbs up and said "I did it".

In the early hours of the following morning he had a heart attack. Then he had another. Then he died.

Newspapers across the world printed stories about his death and, perhaps due to the intensely private way his family had handled the situation, many reported incorrect facts. One story said the tumour had been removed from his neck, another that he had died on the operating table.

The word **mesothelioma** was barely mentioned and his death was attributed instead, to cancer. [13]

---

[13] Information from Steve McQueen – the untold story of a bad boy in Hollywood by Penina Spiegel (William Collins, Glasgow, 1986), Posters from www.stevemcqueen.org.uk, *Papillion* Press Photo, *The Hunter* lobby card from www.mcqueenonline.com,

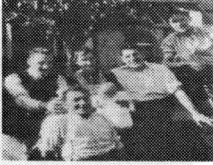

The Standen Family

John and Alice Standen had four sons; John, George, David and Richard (Dick) and two daughters; Eva and Alice.

John Snr

In the 1940's John Standen Snr worked for Newalls Asbestos of Washington, Tyne & Wear as a lagger. He was sent out on contract work and lagged pipes & boilers in factories & buildings around the country. One after the other his sons left school and each spent some time working alongside their father before going off to find other employment as laggers or pipe-fitters.

After a long days work John and his fellow workers went home to their wives and children still wearing the dusty overalls and white-clad dusty shoes. John's daughter-in-law Pat told me

"As T&N did not provide cleaning services for the men's overalls we had to wash them ourselves. I washed Dick's overalls every week. Dick told me some of the men would wear theirs until they practically fell off".

John Snr suffered from thrombosis and died, aged 56, of a heart attack. A the inquest into his death, asbestos was named as one of the factors which contributed to his death.

Eva

His daughter Eva followed him to the grave in 1957, dying of cancer. She was 36 years old.

Then, in the 1970's, three Standen brothers became ill with asbestos related diseases.

* * *

During World War II (1939-1945) the four brothers had joined the navy. John was killed when a troopship he was on was torpedoed off the Italian coast. The others survived. George's war time bride was a local girl named Betty.

David & Else

After the was David went back to being a welder, working with asbestos as part of his daily life. He travelled the world and spent some time in Malaysia where a huge power station was being built. As an asbestos expert, he taught the locals how to handle and use asbestos.

On one of his trips home to England he met the sister of a Danish co-worker. Her name was Else, they got on well and David made a point of visiting her in Denmark.

> "David came to Denmark a few times", she said, "I also went to England to see if I liked it. We were being married. I couldn't speak English!".

They married in April 1957. Else said,

> "Dick and David were so close.. they were like twins. We hit it off straight away. Very well. We would all; Pat, Dick, us, all the kids would go away all together".

Dick & Pat

After being demobbed from the navy, Dick met Pat, whom he married in 1952. He was the first of the brothers to develop an asbestos related disease. Pat tells his story.

> "Dick worked with asbestos right up until when he died. In an early job he mixed up asbestos in buckets and put it on pipes and boilers. He worked in different factories in different boiler rooms. When our kids were young he even worked in a convent".

In 1971 he began to sicken and lose weight. He'd travel home at weekends from his job and, on one occasion, got very annoyed at one of his sons.

"I knew he wasn't right because he was cross with one of the boys and it really hurt me. It just wasn't Dick at all. He loved his boys. He wasn't the kind of man to make a fuss. If he was ill he'd just go off on his own until he was better.

Once he broke a bone in his hand and had to wait a couple of days to get it x-rayed because it had all swollen up. He got up next morning and went to work. In those days if you didn't work, you didn't get paid so he went to work. He nearly passed out. But he didn't like a fuss. That's what he was like.

Dick was taken to hospital and after only a week he was operated on. Then when he was well enough he came home. He had fluid drained from his lungs. He was not well but there was nothing they could do for him. I was told the lining of the stomach was covered in small growths and he had a large stomach tumour.

The Monday before Dick died he was taken into hospital to have more fluid drained off. This was five months after he first went into hospital. He was so thin his bones stuck out. They opened him up and stitched him back up again. There was nothing they could do".

Dick died the following afternoon. He was 46. Pat, at the age of 40, was a widow with four young sons.

"It affected the boys. None of them really knew that their dad was bad. I didn't really know myself. The doctors didn't know.. or said they didn't know. I hadn't told the boys how serious Dick was because no-one really knew how long he would live. I had just told David, my eldest son, the weekend before as I didn't think it could be much longer. So David said he would stay home from work. He was only 16. The other three boys were at my mothers.

I had telephoned the hospital and they said Dick was sitting up having a fight with his lunch.. he was winning or the lunch was winning. He was constantly sick after eating and had been all through his illness. I went shopping and I was going to visit him in the afternoon. It all happened so fast".

Else said,

"Dick was such a shock. I couldn't face him. It was just such a shock. Then George was another shock".

George & David

In 1978 George became ill. He developed pleural mesothelioma, which he suffered from for 15 months. Pat said, "fluid was drained from his lungs. It seemed to be an awful lot".

Sometime in 1978 David hurt himself while playing badminton. "Oh hell, I've busted a muscle", he told Else. Or so he thought. He had a pain in his side. Else tells his story.

"After a week the doctor said that it wasn't a muscle. He sent David to hospital for tests and scans. It was autumn 1978. He was clean. There was nothing on the x-rays or anything.

He was in pain all winter. He was fed up working, working, working and wanted to let us have a bit of a rest. It never dawned on me.

David worked right up to two days before he went into hospital on Wednesday 8th March 1979. It was the last test they could do. To operate. On Thursday afternoon I went to visit. I hardly recognised him. When the surgeon came in I was called out. They were to operate on Monday but the surgeon said "I cant wait. I have to operate right away".

There was nothing in his organs. All clean, nothing on the lungs, nowhere. It was growing in the intestines, between them, like big fingers. One of them burst when he played badminton.

The doctor said there was nothing they could do. He knew David was a clever man and he said "I must tell him because he's too intelligent a man not to be told". David was exceptional, with his brain and his hands. He was always reading. He built our house. He didn't really want to know. He had never been ill. He knew what had happened to Dick.

George was getting injections and David thought, "Oh well, perhaps they've found something they can do with the asbestos". He still thought he could survive.

In three weeks I took him home. Myself. There was an ambulance strike. In five weeks he died, in our home we built ourselves. It was good that I could do that for him. They wanted to put him in a hospital to die but I said 'no thank you'".

In Copenhagen Else had trained as a nurse for newborn babies. She had also spent some time nursing in hospitals and so her experiences helped her to cope with her very sick husband.

"I just got on with it. I didn't think about it. But it was very hard work. I didn't sleep at night. He needed medicine, morphine, every three hours. If it is not your husband you look after then you don't do it. In eight weeks he was only skin and skeleton. To see them go to nothing… you just don't think it is possible".

"It all happened so quickly", Pat said, "It seemed as though if they had been opened up, it acted faster".

Through-out David's illness, George was in hospital and was completely unaware of his brothers suffering. David didn't want him to know. "Keep that away from him", he had told Else, "Give him my love".

David died on the 2nd May 1979 at 11:45pm. On the 3rd, at 8am, George died. Barely eight hours were between them.

On the morning of the 3rd, Else telephoned Betty to tell her of David's death. Betty then telephoned Pat and, as they talked, the hospital were trying to get through to tell her that her husband George had died.

Because Pat had lost her husband Dick just a few years before, the Standen family tried to shield her from the illnesses of George and David. "I didn't know exactly what was going on", she said. "They shielded me a lot from it. So I only got bits of information years later".

When Else tried to claim against her husband's employers, T&N blocked everything. They denied all knowledge of David, even denying that he had ever worked for them. T&N claimed that all their records had been destroyed during the war.

However, Pat found an old tax record belonging to Dick and through this Else was able to recover information from the tax office, which proved where her husband had worked.

The legacy of asbestos meant a fight for Betty. The doctor refused to mention asbestos on her husband's death certificate. T&N also denied all knowledge of George. His case was dropped but later re-opened by his son (who happened to be a doctor).

Chase Manhattan [14], the large New York based company, who were also suing T&N themselves at the time, provided the family with relevant T&N papers so they could fight – and win – their case. Pat said,

"The trial took place in October 1993 with the findings given in March 1994, six

[14] see chapter *Armley, Leeds & Mumbai* and *References*

months later. The judge, who had never dealt with a compensation case like this before, did a very good job"

Ex-work colleagues, and friends, of the Standen family have gone on to developed asbestos related diseases. Several of Dick's ex-supervisors have died over the years due to 'cancer'.

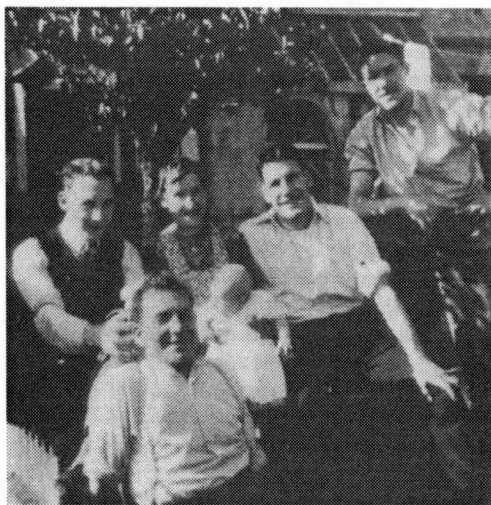

The Standen Family;
David, Alice, George, Dick and John Snr (front) [15]

---

[15] Photographs by the Standen Family

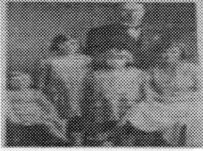

Children Of The Dust

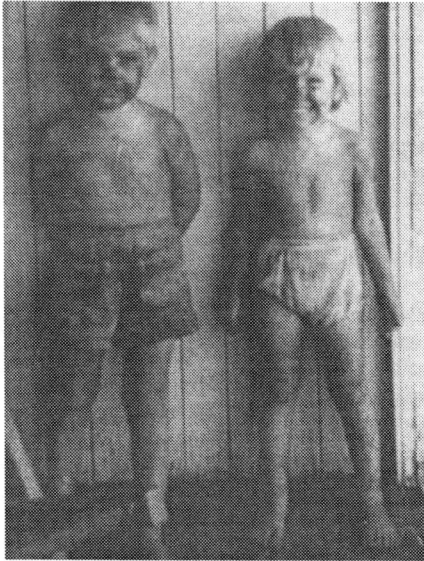

The photograph. Two children standing side by side. On the left is a boy aged about 6 years old. On the right a girl aged about 4, bright smile on her face.

They both look fair but it's hard to tell because of the dirt they're covered in. It's in their hair, on their faces, probably in their mouths. They are barefoot, wearing shorts and their skin is covered; chests, legs, hands, feet, knees.

Normal kids having fun playing and getting dirty. But the horrific thing about The Photograph is the realisation that this 'dirt' is **blue asbestos dust.**

These are two children of Wittenoom, Australia. Children of the dust. They played in it, breathed in it and a visiting doctor was horrified to see them sitting digging in it.

The family. The parents are Philip and Esther. The children are Virginia, Shirley and Val, Philip got a job at Wittenoom and in 1953 his family moved there. Val, the youngest at 13 years old, remembers the dust well. The entire town had a constant blue haze over it. She said,

> "What I remember most from those early years was the heat, the bloody heat. It was scorching. On top of that there was dust everywhere around the town from the tailings they used to dump. It was on the driveways, on the roads, on the basketball court. If you fell over you got filthy. It was in your eyes, your hair, all over your clothes".

The girls grew up and eventually married local men. In time some extended family moved to Perth.

Philip died in 1970 of asbestosis followed six months later by Esther (mesothelioma). Three years later Val's husband died (asbestosis) followed by Shirley's husband (bowel cancer) and Virginia's husband (asbestosis & cancer).

In 1989, at the age of 49, Val died of mesothelioma. The dust she had been exposed to in the town as a child had killed her.

There was no escape from that dust for any child of Wittenoom. Some died in their 20's.

Australia is a rich country. But across the world, poorer countries have habitually used child labour in asbestos mines. In South Africa, in the 1940's, children as young as 12 were discovered to have serious heart damage. They worked in a blue asbestos mine and their job was to trample down asbestos fibres into sacks before the raw material was shipped abroad. The doctor who examined them did not expect them to live long enough for mesothelioma, lung cancer or asbestosis to develop.

From these mines asbestos was shipped all over the world. Dockers in the shipyards unloaded the stuff and unknowingly carried lethal dust home to their families. Raw material went into asbestos factories where it was made into products. Men and women handled it with their bare hands just as they do now, in 2007, in Mumbai, India [16]

John Kennally's mother worked at the JW Roberts factory in Armley and she always came home from work covered in dust. John, a child, was exposed to raw asbestos. He died in 1988, aged 42, from mesothelioma.

Another Armley victim was Nellie Kirby who died at 42 from mesothelioma. Her father came home from the factory in his dusty overalls and hug his children or bounce them on his knee.

Children, exposed to asbestos by parents coming home from work in an asbestos factory continue to die from mesothelioma. Homes had trails of dust, in carpets, on furniture, on clothes.

This is *Trudy McPhillips* story

> "I was born in Washington, County Durham where there was a chemical works and asbestos plant belonging to Turner & Newall. The houses and back streets were covered in white dust and we had a house directly opposite the factory. My father and brother worked there.

---

[16] see chapter Armley, Leeds & Mumbai

But as children we all played amongst this dust. There was also a very large, what we called, a pulp heap, which was all waste from the factory. We played on this too. Our shoes, I remember, were covered with this white pulp, which hardened.

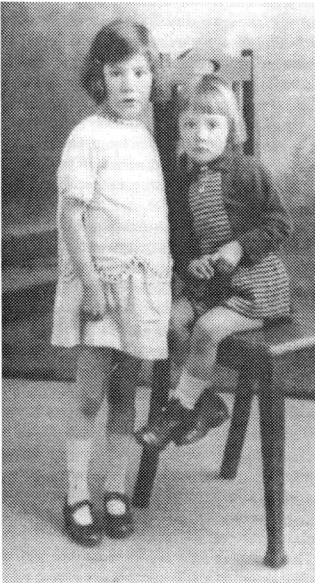

Edna & Trudy McPhillips

Dad and my brother had to shake their clothes and overalls in the back yard, after finishing a days work.. not that it made much difference to our home as everything was covered in white dust.

I didn't leave there until I was 19 years old to be married. I had three cousins and two uncles who died of 'lung cancer'. They too all worked in the same factory.

Masks were never thought to be needed. My father also died of 'lung cancer'"

I met Trudy in 1994. By then she was using a nebuliser three times a day and found her diseases very difficult to cope with. From being very active she could barely get off a bus.

"Sometimes I break down. It's just because I can't do the things I used to. It's unfair.. you're healthy all your life and now, when you should be enjoying retirement.. this".

As a child Trudy had been a tomboy who enjoyed the rough and tumble of play. "We used to run up and down the pulp heap. Great fun", she said. She also clearly remembered her uncles and cousins dying of 'lung cancer'. "They couldn't breath and we tried to open windows to let some air in but, of course, the windows and ledges were all white dust. It was everywhere".

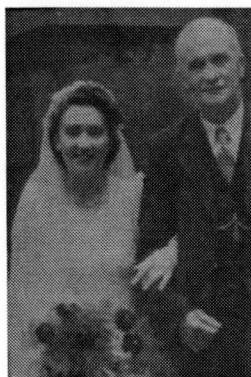

Trudy & her father 1950's

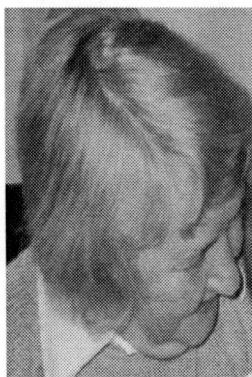

Trudy 1998 [17]

---

[17] Photographs;
McPhillips Family (small insert photo) and Trudy McPhillips & her father by Trudy McPhillips
Dusty children of Wittenoom by Asbestos Diseases Society of Australia
Trudy 1998 by B McKessock

Trudy was a dear lady who welcomed me into her home. I don't know what happened to her as we lost contact some time ago. My letters are cards were, one day, never replied to. I can only assume she has passed away.

Across the UK people live with asbestos every day. In 1991 sixty families were evacuated from an estate in Portsmouth. The estate was built on an old naval rubbish dump.

In 1977 sacks of raw asbestos which was dumped on land beside a nursery. Very young children stood bemused at a piece of rope, watching men in space suits 'safely' remove the dangerous material just a couple of feet away.

Asbestos removal professionals are not always that careful. In Armley, in 1995, a local resident Irene Merrill watched in horror as workmen pulled apart a house, threw things out of the windows and generated dust. She said

> "There were kids everywhere. We have been warned not to disturb any dust.. and here are these men. I explained to one man how dangerous it was, he was very nice, very apologetic. I don't know if I got through to him. People just don't understand"

During the war thousands of gas masks were produced to protect Britain's children in the event of gas attacks. In 1942 a special feature was introduced into some. Blue asbestos fibres. It was thought that the fine fibres would help to protect the wearer against the latest German gases.

Margaret was evacuated from Glasgow at the age of 8. "it was great fun, a big adventure. But the gas masks were terrible. They made this sucking noise when you tried to breath with it on, you couldn't talk properly".

In the 1980's the factory where the masks were made had an epidemic of mesothelioma as former employees (mainly women) began to die. One of the scientists said

"We thought we were saving lives. None of us had any idea we were killing people".

Talcum powder, used on babies' bums throughout the western world, used to contain asbestos. In 1993 a spate of cervical cancers in the south of England were blamed on such talc. How many babies have been exposed, ready to grow up and suffer from an asbestos related disease? Did you or your parents use talc? Are you one of them?

Even the unborn are at risk.

In 1991 an autopsy performed on a full term, still born baby found asbestos fibres in the child's lungs. A baby that had never even breathed a single breath outside of it's mothers womb.

Mum, Me &
Mesothelioma

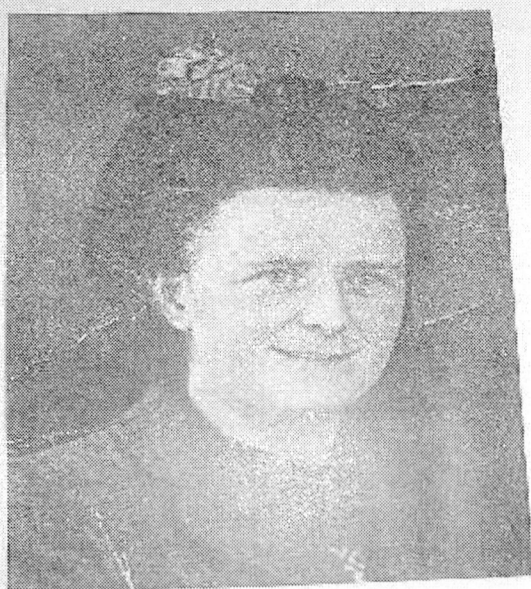

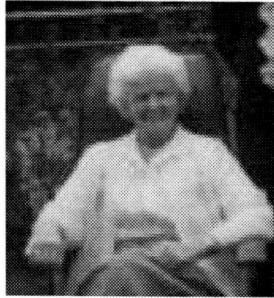

Ellen's Story

In April 1992 my mum, Ellen, felt a pain in her back, which just would not go away. She then spent months going to the hospital for tests to find out what was wrong, why it wouldn't go away and why it was gradually getting worse.

Eight months later, she had a biopsy.

On Christmas Eve 1992 the biopsy results were known.

My mum had mesothelioma.

Throughout 1993 the disease got progressively worse and she spent a lot of time in and out of hospitals and at the Accord Hospice in Paisley.

They tried various treatments but nothing, except morphine to quench the pain, worked.

Eventually she decided she didn't want to live in a hospice, she wanted to come home. My dad, Stan, and I took care of her at home. I gave up my life away from home and returned to take care of her full time.

She spent her final few months at home and, just after midnight on the 6th November 1993, she died in her sleep.

It was eleven days before her 68th birthday.

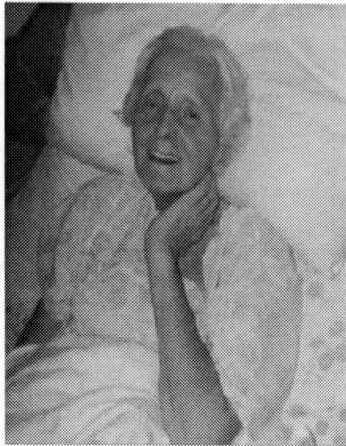

remember remember the fifth of November

I remember the sound of fireworks that night and I remember the sound of fireworks that night, like a ghost coming back to haunt me, every 5th November since then.

Ellen Whitelaw was born in Glasgow in November 1925. She was one of ten children, her eldest sister married and left home so, at the age of 13 when their mother died, Ellen became a little mother to her younger brothers and sisters. The youngest child, who was only two, was adopted by an aunt.

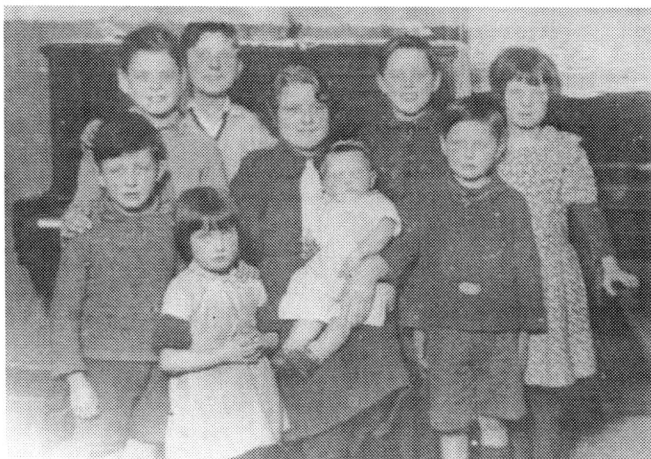

1936 Mums family (she is on the right)

During the Second World War she met my dad, Stanley McKessock. He had joined the navy after being called up. He was serving in the North Atlantic Fleet (The Artic or Russian Convoys) on an aircraft carrier.

The navy accompanied merchant ships in the icy North Sea as they made their treacherous journey into Russia with supplies. It was nicknamed the 'suicide mission'. Over 3,000 men died, the bodies of most of whom were never recovered [18]

---

[18] Additional Information on the Arctic Convoys
http://www.mckessock.com

One night, in 1944, he met my mum at the Barrowlands Ballroom in Glasgow. They had a war time romance and married in 1946.

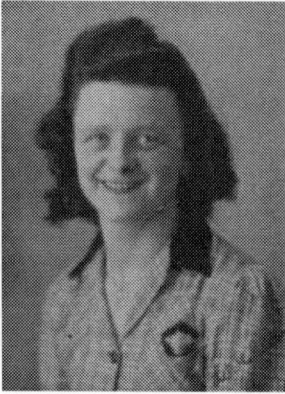

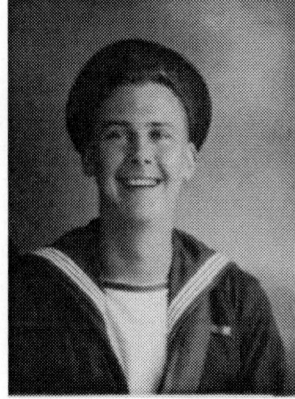

1944 Ellen (the first photo she ever sent my dad) & Stan
He spoke Doric and she couldn't understand a word!

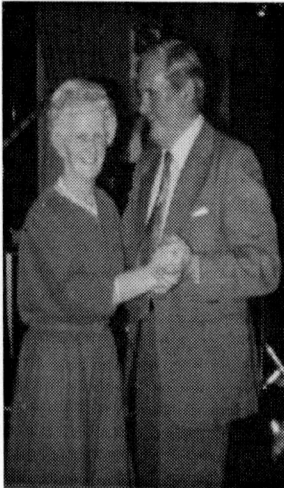

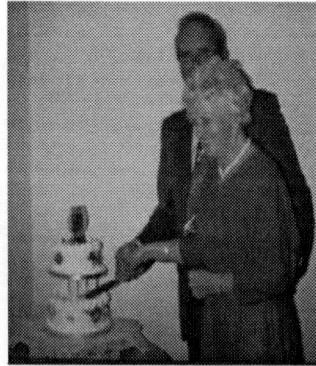

Ruby Wedding 1986

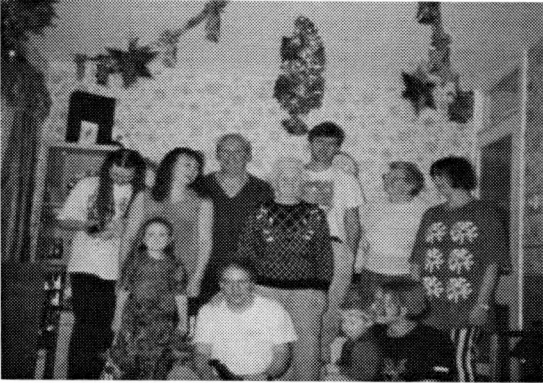

Our Family, Christmas 1991

By the 1990's I had left home and moved north to Perth, Scotland. I still went home every couple of weeks and my parents often drove up to my flat and stayed the night.

Mum had retired and now spent her time at bingo (which she loved) and I was teaching her how to play the piano. She kept active and had a social life with her friends and relatives. At the age of 63 she even learned how to swim.

Whenever I went home mum and me would go shopping in Glasgow. We usually wandered around for a while and I would take her to a pub and buy her lunch and a wee sherry.

So, in April 1992, that's what we were doing. We had parked the car in Glasgow and walked towards the St Enoch shopping centre. Mum complained of a pain in her back but she was determined to ignore it. However half an hour later, she was out of breath and in pain so we decided to go home.

"There's something far wrong with me", she said, "This isn't right".

Concerned, she went to the doctor who suggested it might be a chill or a lung infection. Then he suggested it might be muscular so he gave her a muscle spray. It didn't work.

Mum was then sent to hospital for various tests; x-rays, barium meal, dye in her legs, cameras down her throat, they tried to take fluid from her lungs (painful), a partial biopsy. There were no answers. {see Appendix B - *mums diary 1992*}

In late 1992 I went to see her hospital doctor who assured me that whatever it was, it was not malignant and that they were "keeping a close eye on her". I was unnerved by this, I knew there was something wrong, but what? My mum was never a complainer. If she felt uneasy, I was too. Later that day when I visited her, she told me

"The nurse said I could use the quiet room if I wanted. What did they mean? That's for people with things like cancer, so they can cry". She was upset and puzzled.

There were no answers or any type of information coming from the so-called professionals. What did they suspect? What were they not saying?

In December there were more tests. Mum went around all the main Glasgow hospitals and on the 19th she underwent a biopsy. On the 24th (Christmas Eve) the doctors knew what was wrong.

On the 26th (Boxing Day) my mum's younger sister celebrated her Ruby Wedding Anniversary. Mum drove her car to the party and back. She enjoyed herself but barely danced as she had a fear of someone bumping into her and hurting her back. She was becoming very tender and fearful of people hurting her unintentionally.

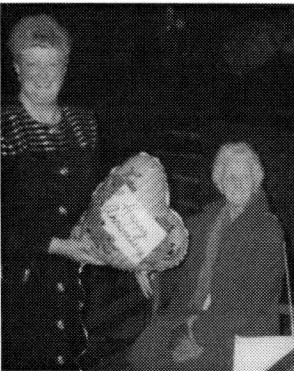

mum (sitting) & her sister

Hogmanay was very quiet affair. My mum always had food and drink ready for anyone who came to the door and she always put on her best dress, make up, perfume and jewellery. She liked to look her best at the bells. But not this year. She couldn't be bothered. After the bells, she went straight to bed. What we didn't know then was that my mum had celebrated her last birthday, her last Christmas and her last New Year.

Early in January 1993, mum and I visited the hospital where we were told the result of the biopsy. Called into Dr Dorwood's office, we sat down as he explained what the diagnosis was.

He said the words 'mesothelioma' and 'asbestos'. We looked at him blankly. My mum had mesothelioma, a tumour in her lung, which had been caused by exposure to asbestos.

Then he asked a question which would later come back to haunt us in a destructive way. "Where would you have been exposed to asbestos?"

Now what you have to remember was that we were both stunned and taking in this information at this point in time. My mum wracked her brains. She remembered using a white board she'd found in her single end (after the war) as an ironing board. As she talked and tried to wrack her memory, In the meantime, Dr D was scribbling in her medical notes.

"Where would you have been exposed to asbestos?"

With hindsight, I would ask why the doctor asked this question?

As a doctor shouldn't he have been more concerned with the emotional and physical state of my mum?

Shouldn't he have been thinking of what care she would be requiring?

Shouldn't he have started discussing what was going to happen next from a medical standpoint?

But no, he scribbled my mums open thoughts on her medical notes. There it was, in black and white - *white board found after the war .. ironing board* - written by a 'professional' person, a 'senior' doctor, a medical 'expert'.

My mothers work history was unknown to Dr D. He did not know that she had worked for a factory that was proven to be full of asbestos. None of that was scribbled in the medical notes.

There is a certain power that people have over others. It is well known. The power of the Doctor over the Patient. And that power can be abused. In our case it was. For whatever reasons that man had, he scuppered my mother's legal case against the people who had exposed her to asbestos. *With one sentence.* A sentence scribbled down from the words of a woman in shock, a woman who had less than ten minutes to recall a lifetime of over 65 years.

We were still stunned when we left that office and I, for one, wanted to know everything I could about mesothelioma.

I'd heard of asbestos, but mesothelioma? What exactly was going to happen? I immediately went in search of information, surfing the Internet, trying to find other people who might know something, visiting libraries, pulling out medical books, anything. My research gave me an idea of what it was and what was to come. My parents didn't have a clue. As my mum asked me questions, I answered her as best I could. She wanted to know the truth.

By March she had what seemed to be a lump on her side. There was a tumour in her right lung and this was where most of her pain was. Medical staff told us the nerves in this area were irritated and causing the pain. Eventually they tried treatment to numb the nerves to relieve the pain.

April was the last time she went to the supermarket. She was too tired, breathless and in pain to do anything but sit down. She never went again.

On the 28th April I took her to the Accord Hospice in Paisley. She had been reluctant to go initially but, as it was just for the day and she didn't have to go again if she didn't like it, she decided to give it a go.

"They gave me a brandy and put me to bed", she said. She liked it!

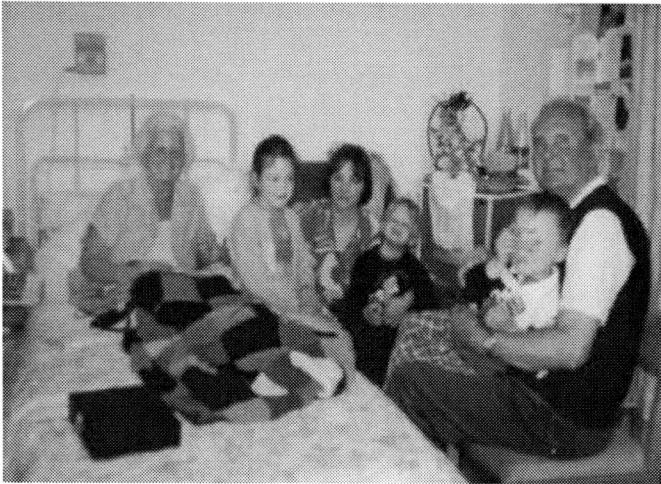

The Hospice May 1993

We spent most of the summer driving her to and from the hospice. Driving her anywhere was a nightmare. She was in pain, her back was sore so we always had to have lots of cushions and pillows for her. I can remember one day driving along, my mum in the front passenger seat surrounded by pillows and cushions. I had to take my time as every bump, pothole or movement of the car caused her agony. So I drove along the quiet back streets in third gear, doing less than 30 miles per hour.

And there is always one, isn't there? A restless driver who comes zooming up behind you, gets irritated at the slow speed you are doing, decides to pass you in a temper and blows their horn at you just to let you know what a bad driver you are.

Could they not see the frail woman in the passenger seat? Could they not see all the cushions & pillows? Could they not use their brain and think 'oh there must be something wrong here?' No, of course not. They were too stupid to put their brain in gear.

My language sometimes was not very polite (to put it mildly!), but my priority was my mother, her comfort and, to be honest, I didn't give a damn what some drivers thought. We were on the back roads and taking our time for a very good reason. If they were too stupid, impolite or impatient that wasn't my problem.

Giving her a hug or a cuddle was another gently-does-it experience. You couldn't actually touch her back with your arms, just pretend to. Unfortunately one member of her family, excited and tearful after seeing her for the first time in years, arrived at our house and gave her a great big bear hug. He crushed her in the process and the pain she experienced was excruciating. I had already explained to him how ill she was but I didn't realise he would hug her like that.

His actions caused her untold suffering for days and she cried, she was confused as to why he had hurt her. Naturally he was upset too when he realised what he'd done. I could see the look in his eyes, 'I'm sorry, I didn't mean to'.

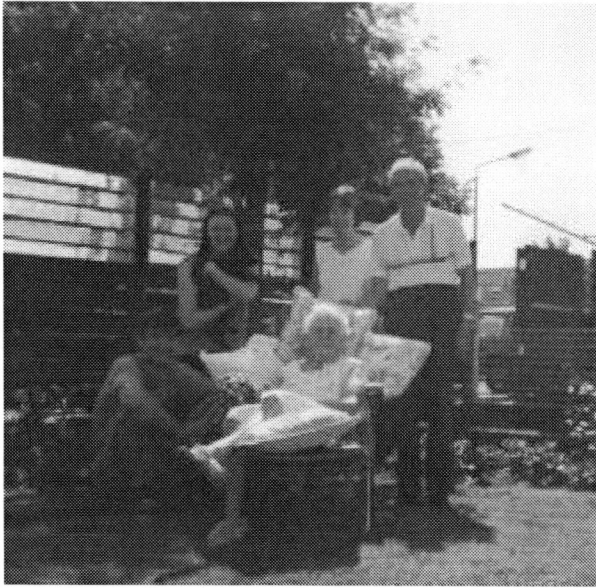

In the garden, summer 1993, mums back being protected by cushions & pillows

Over the next few month's mum spent long hours on the telephone talking to her relatives, desperately looking for support and comfort. Often she never got it. Some of her family, whom she loved, ignored her for a long time. In my mind I tried to understand why. Perhaps they just couldn't cope? As a family, my sisters, dad & mum coped well, at least on the surface. But the strain was always there, quietly lurking under the surface.

In spring 1993 I went for a meal in a restaurant, a special treat for me, given by my boyfriend. I saw two old ladies, about the same age as my mum, sitting chatting. I burst into tears. The realisation that I'd never be able to take her for a pub lunch again hit me hard.

Tears are a release, everyone needs to cry sometimes. It's something I rarely did all my life, it's very unusual for me and it's something I did, usually in private, throughout 1993. However much to my embarrassment (and to whoever I was with) I would sometimes be totally overwhelmed with grief. It didn't matter where I was.

Mum cried too but never in front of us. She would tell me sometimes that she "had a wee greet this morning".

The one great sadness she had was the realisation that she would never know my children. I had a boyfriend but we had no plans to get engaged, married or have kids at that time. I consoled her with the thought that I had photographs and video of her and they would know her through me, and all the silly stories I could tell.

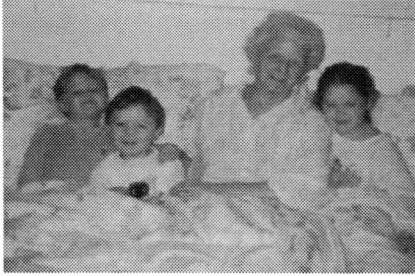

with three of her grandchildren May 1993

Not only was there grief & sadness there was also the anger. Then pent up frustration and violent anger which was gradually building up inside me. It was against the world but when someone got in the way, it would be targeted at them.

'You always hurt the people closest to you' was something my mum would say. It was true.

My poor boyfriend was the target in more than one incident. And yet he put up with me. I became the target for my mother's sisters. The anger might fade but even after all these years, I know it's still there. I hate the people responsible for my mums suffering, which I still remember.

For eight weeks my mum lived at the Accord Hospice where she received the best care and attention the staff could give her. She enjoyed her first Jacuzzi, had her nails painted, her hair done and took part in singsongs in the day room with other patients.

They tried new drugs and combinations of drugs. She suffered from sickness, diarrhoea and the passing of blood. Sometimes she thought she was going to die right there and then.

One day me and dad visited and she told us, "You nearly lost me last night. I thought I was dying. I passed a lot of blood... everything just came away. I honestly thought I was dying".

In June a nerve block operation took place where a specialist tried to numb some of the nerves which were causing her pain. The idea was if it worked they would do another operation to completely kill off the nerves and her drugs could be reduced. It didn't work. Instead she developed a very bad rash all over her back, chest & neck and became ill again.

The Homeopathic Hospital in Glasgow's Great Western Road was where the hospice sent her next for a few days. They thought the treatment may help her. The few days became weeks as she responded to new medicine by becoming ill.

However, she liked the hospital itself. Her bed was beside a large bay window and, aided by a nurse, she could stand and wave 'cheerio' to her visitors.

Mum loved music. It was something that gave her the greatest joy. When she was small she and her brothers and sisters would sing songs around the family piano as their mother played.

Mum put my sister Ellen & I through music school. We played solo's, duets, in groups and in bands and travelled in Europe & Canada with the Jimmy Blair Accordion School of Music. At the National Accordion Championships, when I was about 15, I came 7th in the Junior Solo and Ellen & I went on to win the Scottish & British Duet competitions. Later we won the British Group along with Gary Blair, Ian Duff & Colin McKee.

A lot of us grew up with the Music School. Ellen had started when she was 11, then myself when I was 7. Mr Blair was like an Uncle to us and the parents ran the committee, which gathered funds to subsidise buses, tours and trips to competitions.

Mum became known as Mrs Apple Pie because she'd bake apple pies on a Sunday and bring them along to band practise for everyone. On a Tuesday evening, which was Theory Of Music night, she'd bake a pizza and arrive outside the music school where I'd meet her after work. We usually ended up with other people from the music school in the car, waiting until the class started at 7pm and having pizza. Everyone loved her apple pies and pizzas and all the young kids, even if they didn't know her name, knew Mrs Apple Pie.

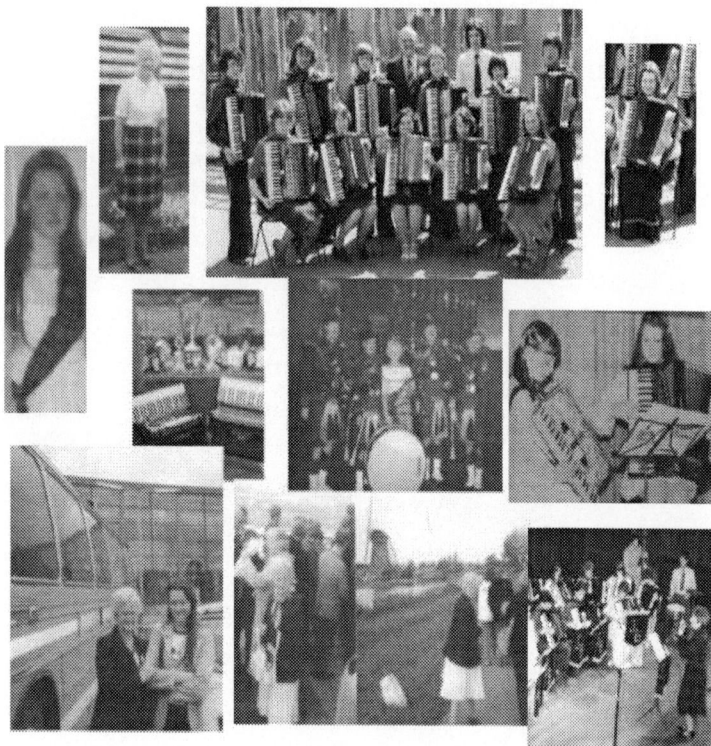

Jimmy Blair Music School
myself (sash), mum, one of the bands (I'm front right, Jimmy Blair is back centre), Ellen, prizes (me & Ellen's), mum with a drum & pipe band we met, me& Ellen, travelling in the Netherlands, Mrs Blair conducting the band

The bands had made a few recordings (I still have a vinyl 45 which was made when I was very young) and mum always had a tape of one we'd made with her (which was pretty embarrassing as she'd put it on in the car no matter who was there, new boyfriend or worse).

So at the hospital one day she decided to brighten things up in her ward. She put the tape on and turned the volume up. Within a few minutes the other patients were jigging up and down the ward to Scottish music, encouraged by you-know-who.

"I got a row the day", she told me. I had all the patients dancing up and down the ward. I put your tape on… they loved it, they were all dancing. And they're supposed to be sick! The nurses came running in and chased them all back to bed. It was good fun. I got a row, it was all my fault". And then she laughed.

Although she liked the hospital, the treatment didn't really do her any good and she was soon back at the hospice. Her condition deteriorated even more and she could no longer wash or dress herself. Dad and I took turns to visit her, he in the afternoon, me in the evening. This way dad got a break and I helped her get ready for bed.

It was around this time that she first let me help her wash and, for the first time in months, I saw her body. It was sickening, she was wasting away. Her legs were painfully thin, she had bedsores on her lower back and there were huge red finger marks where she had been scratching at an itch. There was folds of slack skin around her buttocks where she'd lost fat and muscle. I had to hold my breath and avert my eyes, I thought I'd throw up.

But not once did she see any reaction on my face, she didn't know what she looked like and she didn't know the effect on me. And she never would. It would have hurt her. Every time I washed her I wanted to break down but I couldn't. I waited until I got home. And I wanted to kill. I wanted to kill the people who had done this to her.

Sometimes relatives would visit her and I'd ask them to stay for ½ hour to 1 hour. I became very unpopular, particularly when they ignored me and stayed for two. Inside, I'd get angry at them. They couldn't see what it did to her because they weren't there all the time. Even though she enjoyed the company, it wiped her out. And me & dad had to pick up the pieces and keep our own stressful emotional roller coasters to ourselves.

The cocktail of drugs she was on would often cause her to drift off to some other planet. She got totally stoned. She would become detatched from reality and was easily confused and heavily influenced by what others told her. I jokingly called her a Junkie ☺ and she'd respond by saying "cheeky wee messin", a sly smile coming to her face as she said it.

And she would sing. Lying on her bed with someone beside her, she'd burst into a wee song. Her eyes had laughter in them although her voice was as frail as she was. She lit the room up.

The most important drug was morphine. And she took this in various forms at various stages of her illness. There was sevradol and MST Continus tablets which are both control-release morphine, diamorph which came with a shunt and a needle (which she hated) and oramorph, a liquid morphine. Mum particularly hated the taste of the oramorph and she'd screw her face up in disgust when she knew she had to take it. She said it was "yeuchy, horrible stuff".

In the hospice two nurses always gave her her drugs. They both carried logbooks and every dose & time was systematically recorded. They also had to watch her as she swallowed her morphine, something she didn't understand. She asked them one day why they watched her. Did they think that she was going to give the drugs to someone else? The nurses joked with her and said she might sell it down the town. "Why would anyone wants drugs if they didn't need them?" was her answer.

We used to tease her about being a Junkie, being stoned and having a very expensive habit. The nurses would laugh. She was amused when she had to swallow the yeuchy stuff and I'd say "there goes another thousand quid". A slight, wry smile would appear and in a few minutes she was stoned again.

The dosage of drugs was raised every so often as her body became tolerant. In March she had been on 360mg of MST per day. This had upset her when she first went into the hospice and over heard two other patients discussing their drugs. One was on 40mg, the other 60mg. She kept quiet about it but it preyed on her mind.

In July the dose was up to 1,000mg. MST per day plus oramorph if she needed it for pain, in between getting her timed doses. By August she was on oramorph only and the dose of this by September was 1,800mg per day. By October she was well over 2,000mg.

Morphine, an alkaloid of opium, is one of the most powerful narcotic analgesics. A controlled drug used in palliative care for the relief of pain in the final stages of illness. Put in perspective, another analgesic is heroin.

A relative said to me one day "I hear your mum's on morphine now". My answer was "She's been on morphine for months". It seemed that one she went onto liquid morphine her relatives started to realise the seriousness of her condition.

On top of the morphine, she was on antidepressants, antipsychotic drugs, homeopathic medicine, laxatives and antibiotics. I often wondered how long she could go on before the cocktail, not the tumour, killed her.

At first mum hadn't wanted to come home. She felt safe in the hospice. She had shared a room with two other ladies but, when one of them died, she became distressed. Another lady who then came into the room also died. "Everyone's dying in here", she told me. She was sad, she felt she wanted to come home but it was some time before she finally made up her mind.

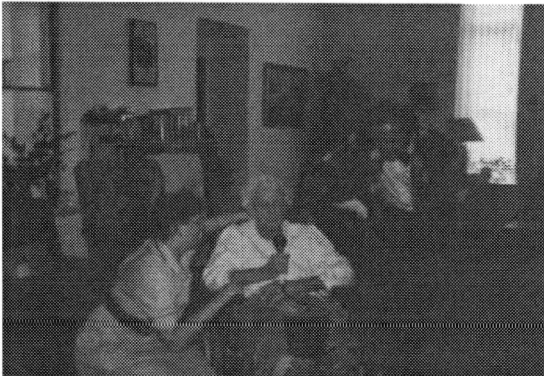

Sing song at the Hospice 1993

(photo by Hospice staff)

One day she awoke to find that someone had placed a vase of white lilies on her bedside table.. Our family always associated white lilies with death, they were the flowers which go with a coffin or placed on a grave. I removed them from the room and realised the staff probably didn't know their significance.

The staff nurse, Maria, discussed mum coming home with me and dad. She knew home was the best place and also knew that mum was unsure. I soon discovered the reasons behind her reluctance. She was afraid that she would be a burden. Another fear was that if she died at home, dad or I would find her.

But home was where she wanted to be and home was where she wanted to die. So, in August, home she came.

When we first brought her home she slept in her own upstairs bedroom. The distance between her room and the bathroom was about 20 feet and gradually, as she became more breathless, this was too far for her to walk.. I would bathe her but soon she couldn't get in or out of the bath. So we resorted to sponge down washes or bed baths.

The most distressing part was her pain. Sometimes, when the effects of her drugs were wearing off, she would cry out. She had set doses of oramorph for set times and in-between smaller doses if she needed them. There was a pattern of acceleration. The more she needed, the quicker her body tolerated it. The other side of the coin was that the more drugs she had, the quicker she would die.

She would cry and beg to be helped.

"Take the pain away".

"Help me, make it stop".

When it's someone you love and you're left with their life literally in your hands – a vicious circle of drugs, pain, death – what do you do? You do your best.

It was around this time when her panic attacks began. Getting to the bathroom was an ordeal and by the time she'd walked back to bed she was desperately gasping for air. Thinking her lungs were going to pack up completely, she'd panic.

I was the only person who could calm her. I would breath with her, big deep breaths as much as she could and talk 'nice & easy' telling her she was doing great and keep going. Eventually after 20 minutes or more, she would relax and her breathing, stilted as it was, would get back to normal. If I wasn't in the room with her she'd panic and try to call me, using up oxygen she needed and panicking more.

Getting up and down the stairs became too much for her and eventually she was trapped in her room. The hub of activity was in the living room so, no matter how hard we tried, she became isolated.

We decided to make the living room her bed-sit. A bed was moved downstairs and part of the settee went upstairs. The district nurse gave us the loan of a chemical toilet and, using the large living room cupboard, we created her own en-suite toilet.

Getting her down the stairs was a challenge. She couldn't walk, my dad was afraid he'd drop her so I offered to carry her down. She was scared I'd drop her and asked for my boyfriend to carry her instead. He's a strong man and I knew she'd be okay. So he picked her up and carried her downstairs, no problem at all.

She liked the new arrangement. She had company and she was comfortable. Knowing she'd be confused for the first few nights I slept on the floor beside her. Once she was settled I went back to my own room upstairs.

I had bought a baby intercom and placed it beside my bed upstairs. With it I could hear what was going on in the living room. Mum had her bell and she'd ring it when she needed anything. It was very effective particularly in the middle of the night!

For a joke she'd ring it "just to see if it's working" or to see "if my servants are listening". She always had a sense of humour!

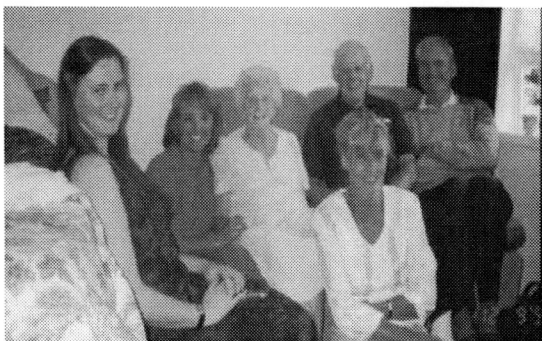

Mum in her white nightdress sitting beside her big brother Tom who came over from Canada to see her. Her bed (on the left) was by now in the living room. Tom died of a heart attack, not long after my mum's death.

One day she asked me "Am I going to die?", "Am I dying?" I was a bit stunned. And I felt sad. I knew the answer was 'yes'. She was lying in bed, I was fixing her covers. She already knew what I might say but it was as if she wasn't sure if I'd tell her the truth. The truth she already knew.

She just had to hear it spoken out loud. She wanted to know. I looked her straight in the eye and quietly said "yes mum, you are". She said nothing and I sat with her for a while. I remember thinking "what do you do when you're life is at an end? What do you think? What would I think?"

The most frequent visitor was her sister Margaret who came to the house almost every day. She had taken good care of mum throughout her illness, visiting her in hospital & hospice and bringing cakes and goodies for a cup of tea. She washed my mums nighties and told her all the latest gossip.

Other relatives, as they began to realise how ill she was, began visiting more often. But others were still confused. One of them, delighted at the news that mum was home, told my sister that it was good that mum was better and out of the hospice. My sister replied "She's not better, she's home to die".

Another relative who had came up from England for a family wedding apologised to me for not visiting her. I'd gone to the local pub to say hello to him and there we sat. He said he'd visit her 'next time'. Angry and frustrated I thought 'there wont be a next time'.

Looking after someone all day, every day is a very tiring, stressful experience. Sleep patterns are disrupted and sleep itself becomes interrupted and fractured. Responding to mum's bell early one morning, I fell down the stairs. It was du to tiredness. Dad became irritable over minor, unimportant things. On one occasion we ended up screaming at each other over…. a pot of mince!

However the most important person was mum and in the last few weeks of her life, dad was the most patient, kindest man in the world to her.

Often she'd sit and stare into space, unaware of what was going on around her. What was going through her mind? What was she seeing? At other times she was witty and sharp, a glimmer of who she really was.

Her biological clock was distorted and she'd want things at odd hours of the day or night. Time meant nothing to her. When she came home to stay, my dad and I took care of her 24 hours a day, 7 days a week. It was demanding and stressful. I'd usually do the night shift, dad did the day shift but sometimes we did both.

Her illness made sure we were always busy and often, in the middle of the night, I'd have to explain that it wasn't dinnertime but would be breakfast soon.

She had a bell beside her bed and if she needed something she'd ring it. I'd hear it through the baby alarm by my bed and respond. On one of those nights she had me up at 4am. She wanted company and decided a wee sherry would be nice. Alcohol alongside all her drugs? Who was I to argue. Anything she wanted, I gave, and a wee sherry was nothing to the morphine. I also knew she liked the thought of a wee sherry.

On my return from the kitchen, sherry in hand, she was asleep. I went back to bed. Half an hour later the bell went. Where was her sherry, she demanded? I had to laugh. The pair of us ended up sitting up to the early hours of morning, mum with her sherry and me with a glass of wine. It was one of the sweetest, and tired, nights I had.

In mid September mum's right eye began to close. She could barely see out of it and the pupil didn't respond to light. Our MacMillan nurse, Innes, would visit once a week and she provided us with a spenco bed (a full length spongy mattress) for underneath mum's sheets. We also got the loan of a sheepskin from the district nurses and all of this helped to ease her painful bedsores.

I had bought her a cushioned ring, which she used for small periods of time when she sat up. Unfortunately a young nurse rather dramatically informed us "we don't use them any more. They do more harm than good". To us the ring helped mum and we only ever used it on occasion. She was dying and if it relieved her of her pain for a little while, was it wrong? But, because she'd heard the comments, she became reluctant to use her ring again and had to be gently coaxed – without it she couldn't sit in a chair at all.

The hardest thing in the world is to watch someone you love slowly die. In the last two weeks of her life I watched her mentally and physically deteriorate at a rate so alarming no one in our family could quite believe it.

Before our eyes she went from a fun-loving, strong-willed woman to a baby who needed everything done for her. Finally she was like a living zombie, not really with us. And we couldn't stop it.

In the summer of 1993 we had resolved the question of 'more painkiller if it was needed'. Mum had decided herself that if she was in pain, if she needed painkiller, if it would put her over her dose – even if it killed her – she wanted it.

The decision was hers and hers alone and, realising that one day she may not be able to make that decision for herself, she made her wishes clear to us, her family.

The most important thing was that she shouldn't suffer. My dad and I strove to make her as happy and comfortable as possible. We knew she was dying. She knew she was dying. What was the point of denying her drugs when she needed them? Especially when, if by doing so, we prolonged her agony. By October she had very little quality of life. She didn't want to live, she was just hanging on.

By now the only time she got out of bed was to use the bathroom. She needed help for that too. Each day a district nurse would visit and, because of the state of her bedsores, the nurse tried applying comfeel dressings on the bottom of her spine. Disorientated and confused, she would pull them off saying "there's something sticky there".

It was like dealing with a small child. I would patiently explain to her what the sticky things were and that she had to leave them alone. Eventually she'd understand and agree to leave them alone. Five minutes later we'd be back to square one "but it's sticky…."there's something sticky there" and she'd be trying to pull them off again. All the understanding had gone.

She always kept her sense of humour – right to the end.

One day she was sitting in bed with something in her hands. Concentrating deeply she sat and folded the object (which turned out to be Ellen's new black velvet hat). I asked her what she was doing?

"Folding"

"What are you folding?"

"Folding, folding"

"What is it?"

"Folding. It's a wee bag. A wee bag."

"It's not a bag, it's a hat"

"No, it's a bag"

"It's a hat. A velvet hat. It's Ellen's"

"Is it? I'm Ellen"

At this point we showed her it was a hat and put it on her head. She was delighted with herself.

"Take my picture then"

So we did.

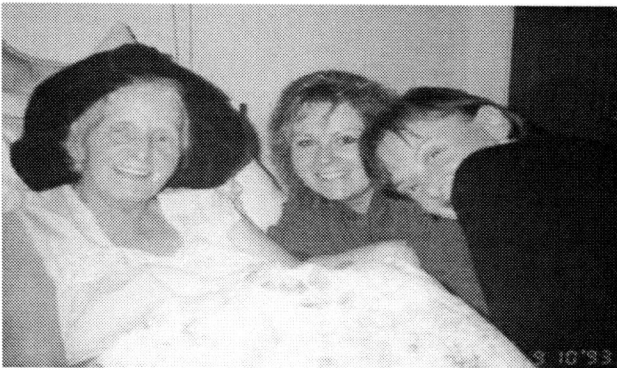

Mum, Ellen & Anne 1993

She once told me "If only I had 10 more years. Just 10 more years. Then I would have died content".

She was staring death in the face and she knew it. Our local doctor was quite religious and sometimes he'd say a little private prayer with her. It seemed to calm her.

In the last two weeks of her life her condition had deteriorated so badly that thoughts of euthanasia and mercy killing went through my mind. Yes, I thought it. I wondered what would happen if I put a pillow over her face, let her out.

Watching her suffer was almost unbearable. I would often sit beside her and think about it. But I felt I didn't have the right, or maybe I just wasn't strong enough. I don't know. I wondered if other people in similar situations had thought the same and would they even admit it to themselves let alone anyone else?

By now she couldn't walk to the bathroom even though we'd moved the bed right beside the cupboard. Dad would lift his 'frail wee wifie' (as he called her) up and carry her there and back.

Swallowing became a problem to her and we had to be very careful not to give her anything that could make her choke. She completely lost her appetite coaxing her to try to eat was a long time-consuming process. I had to time when I thought she'd wake up so that I had something ready for her. Putting it in front of her and spoon-feeding was the only way I could get something into her stomach. A baby cup was bought so that she could enjoy a cup of tea without spilling it. Gradually she came off solids completely and went onto liquids – the reverse of what a baby would do. She was going backwards.

Simple things like getting fresh sheets on her bed gave her the greatest pleasure. It became a knack to change the bed while she went to the bathroom, carried there by dad. I would strip the bed, turn the spenco over, get the sheepskin on followed by towels, sheets, pillows, blankets. By the time she was ready to get back in it was all nice and fresh. Climbing back in she'd coo "This is lovely, this is great".

The towels under the sheets became necessary when her bedsores got really bad. One sore was huge, at least 3 inches long, and it would sometimes bleed. She couldn't lie in any other way except on her back so her spine became a pressure point and more sores followed. There was no flesh to separate the bone from the skin so the sores got progressively worse.

On Tuesday the 2nd November the doctor paid us a visit. For a few moments they were alone and they said a little prayer. He informed us that her lungs were filling up with fluid and she had "maybe a week left". After he had gone she said to me

"My eyes are full of water. Fix them tears".

The next day I sat on my knees beside her bed and spoon fed her runny custard. She had forgotten how to use a straw (again) so I re-taught her. When she finished her custard she smiled and told me to "tell Bobby that was great". Confused, she was convinced that she'd just eaten a bowl of soup made for her by her brother.

At 2am on the morning of Friday 5th November, I heard her making a weird noise. Her words would no longer form and she'd often cry out in her sleep. This time she was trying to call out 'help' (or was it 'hurry', her two favourite words). It was like trying to communicate with a new born baby.

She wanted a drink but was unable to use a straw. Using a syringe I sprayed some water into the side of her mouth. Her mouth, constantly open as she gasped for air, was always dry and we'd spray synthetic saliva (which she thought was wonderful stuff). Calmed, she dozed off again.

For half an hour all was quiet, then she started to call out again. Attended to by dad she fell asleep. At 7.30am we were doing it all again.

At lunchtime my sister Anne helped the two district nurses who had came to change the dressings. Mum was unconscious and they pulled her this way and that to wash her. She didn't know what was going on and she made no noise or response to them.

Her eyes were vaguely open but, at this point, I was sure she was almost, if not completely, blind.

The nurses knew that she would not be with us for much longer and, although they were upset, they tried to break it gently to us. I think, looking back, I blotted it out or I was too tired to think.

Some photographs had arrived that morning from my cousin. One of them, taken in 1979, had the two of them wearing mini kilts, tartan bunnets and singing. We laughed as we passed them around and mum, knowing there was a joke, smiled weakly to join in the fun. It was 3pm. I sat by her and talked, by now I knew she had no sight. I held her hand and I'm sure she didn't even know who was in the room with her. She fell asleep.

By 8pm she hadn't stirred.

By 11pm her throat was making a strange wailing noise. Was this the death rattle?

The doctor arrived, looked at her and said "I think this is her last night.. I doubt if she'll wake up". The week before she'd told him that she was at peace and ready to go. We were not to worry, she'd be okay. In her deep sleep she could not feel or hear anything.

She died, still asleep, in the very early hours of 6th November.

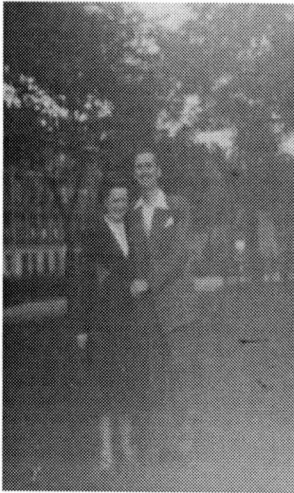

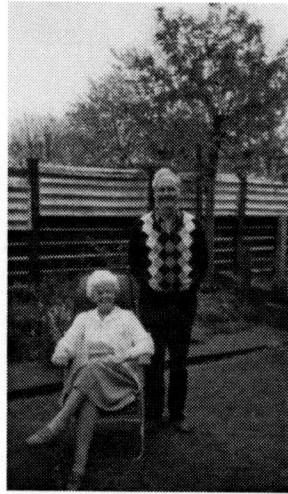

mum & dad, together for almost 50 years

After mum died my dad stayed in Erskine for a couple of years. He built a little shrine to her right by his chair, in the fireplace, putting up photos of her and a copy of the book I wrote.

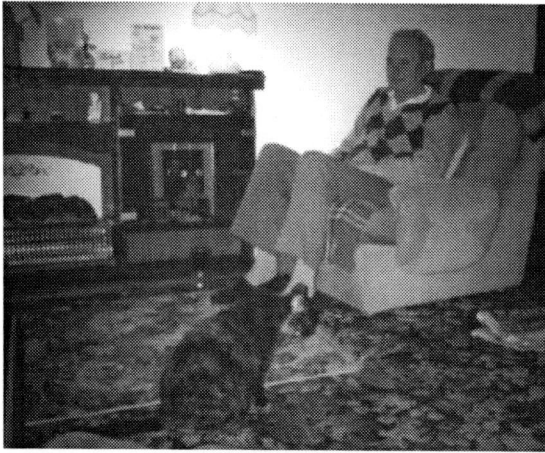

Then one day in 1997 he broke down and told my sister Ellen how desperately lonely he was.

At that point we sold the house and my boyfriend (by now my husband) hired a van, he and Ellen cleared out the house, and he & some of his belongings were taken to my sisters house where he now lives. He frequents the local pubs where he's well known and we all get together now and again at one of our houses, usually at his birthday or at Christmas.

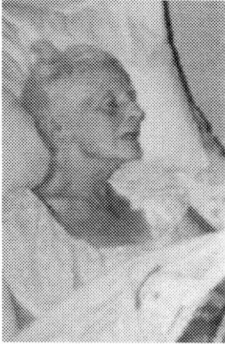

Death & Dying

She asked me "Am I dying?"

I answered

"Yes mum, you are"

Thinking back to 1993, I sometimes wonder if my mum had a good or a bad death?

She wanted to be at home.

We took her home.

She wanted her family around her.

We were around her.

She did not want to be in pain.

She wasn't in pain, at least as far as we could make out, she was doped up to the high heavens!

She had discussed her funeral, her purvey and her last wishes. I had always listened to her and let her take control of any conversation relating to anything she wanted to talk about, particularly her death and what she wanted to happen after it. We were open and honest with each other and it comforted her. The result was also that she told me things about my own family that I had never heard before, some things personal to her.

In the last few days of her life, I used to watch her lying in her bed. She gazed at the wall in front of her. For hours. When I spoke she didn't seem to hear and she didn't seem to see. Regardless of that, I still talked away to her and involved her in the conversation.

On the day she died, I couldn't rouse her from her sleep. I had talked to her in the morning, given her the pills and had tried to turn her over. Her bedsores were awful. She had wailed at me , like an injured animal, because it hurt. I stopped. I just couldn't turn her over, physically it hurt her, and emotionally it hurt me. I had to leave the room.

When the nurses arrived her sores distressed them. They were blue and the room stank. Was it gangrene? The smell of death? It was November but we had opened all the windows. We had to. The nurses changed her bed, helped by my Anne. They were sad and said she had very little time left and they didn't know if they were coming in tomorrow.

Dad gave her medicine in the afternoon then she slept. From that moment on nothing could wake her. In the very late evening I eventually telephoned the doctor who said this may be her last night. With hindsight I should have realised she was never going to awaken, but was I in shock? Was I too tired? Was I denying it to myself? I don't know.

That night we watched a film. She had slept for hours. At the end of the film, Anne & I went upstairs to bed. Through the baby alarm I heard my dad moving about. Something strange came into my head, I sat up. He switched off the TV. And there it was.

Silence.

There was no breathing. That noise I had lain awake night after night listening too, that noise which was ingrained in my subconscious. It had stopped.

Then I heard him calling us.

We rushed downstairs, we knew she'd gone, yet it was as if we didn't believe it. It was strange.

Anne looked at her and said "poor wee mammie".

She had died in her sleep. There was no trauma.

She had just stopped breathing. The tumour had finally strangled her lungs. Her medication had kept her asleep.

I was relieved. Yes I was. She was out of pain.

It was the early hours of Saturday morning. The funeral directors came and took her body away.

My sister Ellen was arriving on a train and later in the afternoon my dad and Anne went into Glasgow to get her. I wandered around the house and I remembered my neighbour, Donald Sinclair (a boy I had known since Primary School), saying "if there's anything I can do". So I went to see him.

He was fantastic. He moved mums bed back upstairs for me (big strong lad!), we moved the furniture in the living room around, he went home (I hope his back is ok), I put the dinner on and went for a shower. And there I was when I heard them coming home and the voices… "oh my god, what's she been doing….. **and** the tea's on…". When I came out they refused to let me help, sat me down with a glass of wine and told me to stay put. We laughed.

The strangest thing seemed to occur after my mum's death. It was as if a big relentless burden had gone. The burden of watching her in pain, of trying to make it ok every day and night, of seeing her deteriorate and being unable to stop it. It was a huge relief.

A day or so before the funeral we decided to take dad to a local pub for lunch. Mums body was at the funeral home, I had telephoned all her relatives to let them know that if they wanted to visit her, they could. Just before we set off to the pub one of our cousin's arrived at the house. It must have been bizarre for her.

There we were, smiling, joking, going to the pub and our mother had just died? We were mourning but we were also relieved. Unless you have felt that relief, you will never know. It cannot be described.

Before she died, she and I had discussed what she wanted at her funeral. She brought the subject up herself and I listened and talked to her.

She wanted a piece of music played *Cavaliera Rusticanna* and she didn't want boring old hymns and people crying. She wanted everyone to have a drink at the purvey and for everything to be nice and happy.

My mother's funeral was lovely. It really was.

The minister had came to our house and had talked to us about her. The sermon he gave was a celebration of her life. It was funny, witty and summed her up perfectly. How she'd pinched my bike off me when I was 13 and left me with her shopping as she rode away, daft things like that, that she had done.

The crematorium was packed. I had spoken to people outside before we went in and I had been fine. I listened to the background music as people came in and I was fine. But when they brought he coffin in, I lost it. I have never cried so hard or shook so much in my life.

Mum in a box those were the words in my head. My boyfriend, not knowing what to do, put his hand on my back then took it away again, fearing he'd make me worse. His instincts were right, though, I needed support.

The music she picked sounded lovely. It was a very unusual, 'good' cremation, if ever there was such a thing. I think she would have approved. With the state I was now in, when the funeral was over I went straight outside and into a car. We had thought about lining up to shake people's hands (as some families do) but I was in no condition. I have no idea if my sisters and dad did, I think so, but I can't even remember. I just wanted to escape.

The purvey was held at a pub in Clydebank, one my dad had picked. We had gone to see several but the final choice was his. He didn't want anything too conservative and the place we went to was more like a pub/bistro, with a long bar. It was nice. Everyone got a drink when they arrived and they did a buffet for us; plates of sandwiches, sausage rolls, cake, etc, the usual, which they took to each table.

After a while we, the close family, decided to split up and go around to thank everyone for coming. My dad wasn't really up for it so we left him in good company, with a pint & a whiskey and me and my sisters all went off in different directions.

As I walked towards the corner I had been allocated, two of my aunties and a cousin came towards me. I will never forget their first words to me…*"we never got any sausage rolls"*, *"we never got any sausage rolls"*, "they *never got any sausage rolls"*…

My mother was dead.

This was her funeral.

My mother's family's words
to the grieving were…

"we never got any sausage rolls".

I was too stunned to reply.

There is a very heavy, emotionally draining burden, which falls upon anyone who has to take of someone who is dying. At the time I didn't realise it, I just got on with it. My aim was to make my mum comfortable and to keep her happy for as long as she had.

My family were all married with children and jobs. I was a student. I had no job, no house, no kids. So when she needed someone at home, it was me who went home to help my dad. There is no way he could have handled it all alone. With my life on hold, I operated, sometimes, like a zombie.

Day after day, night after night, broken sleep, laughter, tears, total relentless mental and physical exhaustion all took its toll on me.

At the time, when she was having a sleep, my boyfriend would take me out for a walk. We never went very far just over the hill and down to the Clyde then back again. When he wasn't there I spent all of my time in the house.

After my mothers death it took me years to regain normality or at least to appear normal (whatever that is). But the emotional roller coaster of bereavement would hit me at any time, night or day, in any situation.

I would be sitting in a pub and see two white haired ladies having lunch. I'd think of her and realise she'd never do that again. My poor boyfriend who'd gone to the bar to get us a drink would return to a crying, emotional wreck. Any white haired lady wearing a red coat, walking along the street, would set me off. And there were a few of them.

Depression, the dark pit of nothingness set in and the long suffering boyfriend would, yet again, try to take me out for a walk; local parks, a wander around the town, museums, anything to try to lift the mood. We tried to just get on with life and resume where we had left off. We went to concerts, pubs, cinemas, everything we had done before, yet I was an emotional mess. I didn't try to fight it, I just went into zombie mode, yet again. It would eventually pass, wouldn't it?

All this time I needed someone to help. I needed the lawyers, our lawyers, to handle my mum's case. I needed them to get on with it and not bother me. I was spent, emotionally drained. I just couldn't be bothered any more.

Funerals and cremations in the years since her death have had a much deeper impact on me. As soon as I see a coffin, I lose it. Not as much as I did at her funeral but, considering I rarely cry, it's bizarre. It's as if I go straight back to that day and that moment in time. *Mum in a box.*

Years before when my Uncles James & Sammy had died I had gone to their cremations. Uncle James had been my mother's favourite brother, something she blurted out when, in shock, she learned of his death. He was a lovely man.

My Uncle Sammy had been my favourite Uncle. He was the one who would tell me stories when I was really young so I'd go to sleep. He had a magic flying jacket (I didn't believe him but it sounded good!). At their funerals I had been sad, but I had held it together. After my mum's funeral, however, things changed. It was as if the full impact of 'the box' really hit home.

When my Uncle Bobby died I had gone to his cremation and I walked past the funeral car and his coffin. I glanced at it and nodded to my cousins. Inside I stood near the back. Everything was fine. Then the coffin came in. *Mum in a box, Uncle Bobby in a box,* and I lost it. Bizarre.

In December 2005 I discovered a family friend of mine was dying of cancer. I had known the family since Primary School, as kids her daughters and I were friends. After we all left Secondary School and we'd all moved on we mostly lost touch. But I'd go back to Erskine and visit the parents; Mr & Mrs McLean. We would spend a Friday or Saturday night having a gin and talking, putting the world to rights. We talked about everything and anything and they always made me feel welcome in their home. I loved them to bits. And now, Mrs McLean was dying.

My mother never got to my Wedding. Mrs McLean did. My mother never got to see my children. Mrs McLean did.

In fact she sometimes briefly watched them for me. They loved the McLean's dog Benji, a big lump of a friendly mutt that made them laugh. The McLean's had rescued him from a dog shelter. To have got the home of Mrs Mclean who loved dogs and long walks, he was a very lucky puppy!

I went to see her as soon as I heard the news. It was strange. There I was, back in Erskine at a house I felt like I practically grew up in.

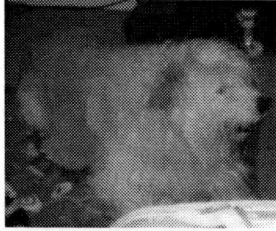

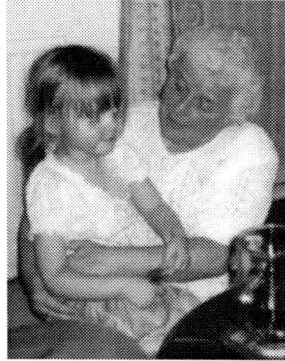

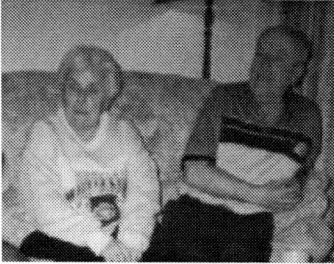

Benji the mad mutt (he was gorgeous), Mrs Mclean with my daughter, Mrs & Mr Mclean

I knew the full well the impact of what being so ill would have on Mrs McLean and her family. I remembered what I had said to people all those years ago when they came to visit my mum. I would ask them, nicely, not to stay too long because it was draining and she couldn't cope. She'd act like she was ok but she wasn't. And, when they'd stayed too long, I would have to pick up the pieces.

Margaret, Mrs McLean's daughter, who had came home from California to nurse her (and still one of my best friends) said she was sleeping so we sat in the kitchen and had some wine. And talked.

After a while I knew I'd have to leave but I really wanted to see her. I just knew that I'd never get the chance again. Upstairs I peeked into her room and saw she was asleep. I quietly went over to her and gently stroked her hair (as I used to do with my mum). I turned to leave and she woke up. She thought I was Margaret, then smiled when she realised it was me.

I only stayed for a brief few minutes and we laughed and cried. At one point she said to me, "Look, if you're going to cry then hand me those hankies and I'll cry as well". She never lost her sense of humour !

She was obviously seriously ill. And I knew what was going to happen. It was like looking at my mother, that tiny, frail, delicate body but the spirit still intact and fighting.

I went back downstairs and stayed a while with Margaret, it was strange that after all these years we had both ended up in the same position, coming home to nurse a mother and coping with a father who was about to lose someone he'd been with for almost 50 years.

Mrs McLean died, with her family beside her, in January 2006.

I went to her funeral. It was at the Catholic
Church in Erskine. I sat at the back. I couldn't
make out where the coffin was, I couldn't see
it. To be honest I was relieved, I didn't want
to see it.

It wasn't until near the end of the service that
I realised it had been there all along, draped in
a white sheet with candles on top of it. I had
wondered but, not being Catholic, I either
didn't realise or I blanked it out. I don't quite
know which. A coping mechanism? And there
it was. *Mum in a box, Mrs M in a box.* And I
lost it.

In 1995 a Doctor on the Western Isles, who
had lost his mother to mesothelioma, wrote to
me after reading the book I wrote. What he
told me then is true. Mourning, the loss, the
sadness never goes away. It may fade but it is
always there. After all these years, I now know
it's true. And when you mourn again for
someone else you care about, it all comes
flooding back.

Lawyers & Our Case
WD & HO Wills (Imperial Tobacco)

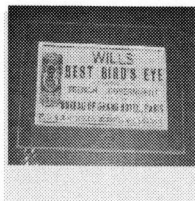

I have never discussed what our case was about and who it was against. I have never written down (except in my diaries) who our family took action against. Not until now. Here it is in black and white.

Everything we, as a family, went through and how it all lead to nothing.

* * * * * * *

We first went to a local solicitors in Renfrew.

We managed to get legal aid and letters seemed to go back and forth every so often. My mum tried hard to remember every aspect of her life; where she had worked, what jobs she had done. Everything. I went over it with her again and again, writing everything down.

Our problem was my mum's memories and to go back to where she had worked decades ago. Finding anyone who was still alive and, most importantly, finding witnesses who could back up what she said was a nightmare.

One of her own close relatives, after saying she would help us, got angry at receiving a lawyers letter and told our lawyer that she didn't want involved.

I was astounded at how many people just would not help in any way at this point in time. One woman was concerned that she'd lose her job if she said anything in a court or to a lawyer. I just kept thinking 'one day this may happen to you, will you want our help then?'. The words 'thanks for nothing' came into my mind a lot.

The solicitors didn't seem to be getting anywhere and, in 1993, we went to a Glasgow firm who specialised in asbestos cases. We had some hope.

My mother had worked for Imperial Tobacco (WD & HO Wills) from the 1960's to the 1980's. They had a factory on Alexandria Parade in Glasgow and my mum worked in the staff canteen. She also, on occasion, took a tea trolley throughout the factory. Asbestos was all over the factory buildings.

Around 1979/1981 the kitchen of the canteen had been renovated. My mum and her colleagues were given new overalls. After her death, I found her white overall with gold stitching, which a friend of mine held into our lawyers. Was it possible there were fibres on it?

Our lawyers lost it. Seriously! They lost her white overall !! How they lost possible evidence was beyond me.

The lawyers had told us Wills would drag their feet. They wanted my mum to die and us to give up. After her death they wanted my dad to die and we'd give up. We took out a family action on behalf of dad, my sisters and myself.

But our legal aid ran out.

In 1995, we were advised by our lawyers to drop the case. The problem now was that if we took Imperial Tobacco to court we, as a family, would be liable for any court costs.

The sentence that the 'professional' doctor had scribbled in her medical report - *white board found after the war .. ironing board* - had been snapped up and used & twisted by Imperial Tobacco. It was implied that the board was white asbestos. There was no proof, of course, it was a technicality.

The doctor's question rang in my head over and over again.. **"Where would you have been exposed to asbestos?"** our stunned confusion at the time, the abuse of professional power that doctor had taken, all of It came to this.

My sisters could lose their homes. My dad could lose his home.

I wanted to fight on, but then I had nothing to lose. For the sake of the family, it was dropped. We never got anywhere near a court and my mothers illness & death were never compensated in any financial way what so ever.

Imperial Tobacco, the firm we had witnesses against, the firm my mother had worked for from the 1960's to the 1980's had dragged their feet for years. Our legal aid was wiped out and we got nothing. Not even the satisfaction of having them publicly named and shamed.

I don't really know where the legal aid went (those lawyers must have written a lot of letters!). It was as if the entire system let us down. I never cared for money, it would never bring my mum back and it would never alleviate her suffering but I wanted people to know who had exposed her and others. I wanted it out in the open. So here it is.

Wills gave annual Christmas parties for the children of staff. So, from about the age of 5, I went to these parties. I was inside that factory along with other kids.

I also visited the canteen on various occasions. I had smashed my teeth when I was 7 and spent years going to the Dentist Hospital in Glasgow. I'd often go and meet my mum at Wills and she'd take me inside. We'd have a cup of tea, her friends were always nice to me. I was probably about 16 or 17 the last time I visited it, possibly older.

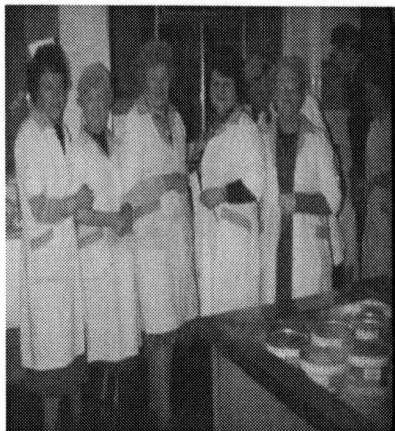

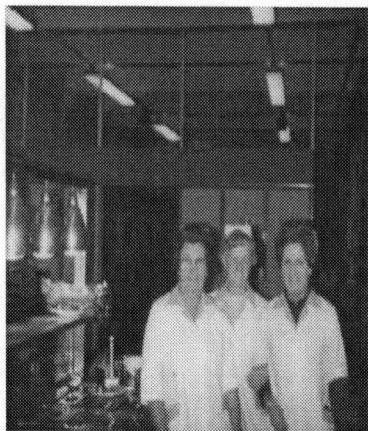

Some of my mum's colleagues in the canteen & mum(right photo in centre) 1979/80 approx

We had testimonies from men who had worked as laggers and who had been inside the Wills factory. One of them told me asbestos was 'all over the place'. I wondered how many of the kids had been exposed? Had I been too? Will time tell?

WD & HO Wills (Imperial Tobacco) Alexandria Parade, Glasgow

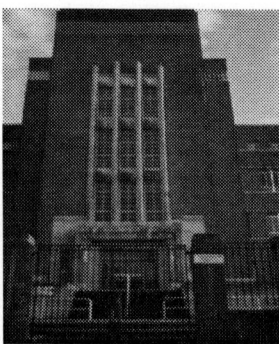

The following are the scanned precognitions
given by four laggers who had worked in the ills
factory at Alexandra Parade, Glasgow which
were taken by our lawyers in 1995

I worked at W D & H O Wills for about 30 years in the warehouse.

The building itself was constructed after the war, probably sometime in the 1950's.

I remember that the pipes were covered with asbestos. I remember the pipes in the basement being covered in asbestos but I cannot remember the situation elsewhere in the building.

I also remember some people coming in to remove the asbestos but I cannot remember when this was. I think it is likely to have been in the 1970's but I cannot remember exactly.

Certainly the factory was quite large and there were a number of pipes running throughout it.

I cannot personally remember any laggers coming in prior to his being removed, but it may well have happened. I remember one occasion when I asked my friend, Jim Wark, who lived on the Parade, whether he was going to come in and do a lagging job that the company was proposing to have carried out. He said that he wasn't, he was doing a job elsewhere, but I cannot remember when this conversation took place. However it certainly suggests that there was asbestos there.

Jimmy Willis

In the 1960's I worked at W D & H O Wills at Alexandra Parade as a lagger. I was sent in as an outside contractor, and I think my employers at the time were Anchor Insulation.

It was quite a long contract that lasted about 3 years. My job was to do the lagging of pipes and boilers. When we first went in there the building was empty. It was under construction as a new factory. We therefore applied the lagging in the usual way that we would with a new building. Then in the last year when we were just finishing off the job, I remember that staff started to come in and work in the factory.

Certainly by the time we left there was a lot of asbestos insulating the pipes and boilers.

Someone I worked with during that time was Jimmy Mulheron and I think also Andrew Rae might have been there but I cannot remember clearly on that.

Martin Moffat

I confirm that I did work at W D & H O Wills during the 1960's.

I was sent in there as an outside contractor to do lagging work.

I was in there for about 2 or 3 weeks. What we had to do was

ventilation work to repair the asbestos lagging on the

ventilation system. This would involve taking off the old

asbestos and then re-lagging it.

There were definitely people working in the factory when we were

there and they did not make any special precautions to protect

them from the asbestos that we were stripping off and applying.

I think that I was employed by Darlingtons at the time.

Harry McCluskey

I used to work as an insulating engineer.

I remember working at W D & H O Wills at various intervals. This would have been during the period 1966 to 1971, although I cannot remember the exact dates.

I remember applying asbestos to the boilers and the factory heating system. I would have used asbestos cloth and rope and also asbestos composition plaster.

We were not given any protection at all at this time, nor was anyone who was working in the factory. The dust would therefore spread everywhere in the factory.

Andrew Rae

NOTE

Jimmy Willis, Martin Moffat, Harry McCluskey and Andrew
Rae gave our family express permission to use their
testimonies in any way against Wills.

We never got to court and there was never any settlement out
of court. Our legal aid – all of it - went on letters to and from
lawyers.

Imperial Tobacco were never held accountable and any
evidence we had, including the above, was never used against
them in any legal form whatsoever.

Imperial Tobacco will, no doubt, claim that there was never
any asbestos in their factory and that they never exposed my
mother or anyone else to it (same story, we've heard it all
before blah blah blah......)

Make up your own mind.

BMcK Jan 2007

Compensation & The Law

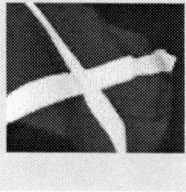

Benefit & Claims

__Industrial Injuries Disablement Benefit__

You __must have__ one of these diseases

1) Pneumoconiosis (asbestosis)

2) Diffuse mesothelioma

3) Primary carcinoma of the lung with asbestosis

4) Primary carcinoma of the lung without asbestosis but where there has been extensive occupational exposure to asbestos__ in specified occupations__

5) Unilateral or bilateral diffuse pleural thickening

NOTE - you don't qualify if
 you were self-employed
or
 you did not develop the disease as a result from your work

or

you developed the disease due to work done before the 5th July 1948

Pneumoconiosis etc (Workers Compensation) Act 1979 Scheme

A lump sum payment to sufferers of <u>certain dust-related diseases</u> (or their dependants if the person has died) who cannot take civil action because their former employers have stopped trading.

Reduced Earnings Allowance (REA)

If you are suffering from an illness or disease, cause by your work, which began before 1st October 1990 and you cannot do your normal work.

There is also **Retirement Allowance** (RA), **Constant Attendance Allowance** (CAA) and **Exceptionally Severe Disablement Allowance** (ESDA).

Leaflets are available through Asbestos Action Groups (who will help you to fill in forms and claim benefits) and through government agencies such as Job Centre Plus.

You will note from the Industrial Injuries Disablement Benefit descriptions of which diseases qualify, *pleural plaques* are not amongst them. Which means that people who have pleural plaques cannot claim the same benefits as those who have other asbestos related diseases.

At the moment asbestos groups are lobbying the UK government to include this disease. Laws have been changed and appealed for the last few years as follows;

The Law

On the 3rd May 2006, on appeal from insurance companies, members of the House of Lords decided that in the cases where a person had been exposed to asbestos (but who had several employers, any one of which could have exposed him or her) the families of the deceased would **not** receive full compensation.

This appeal goes against the judgement they had made in 2002, when the Law Lords ruled that an employer would be 100% liable for exposing a worker to asbestos, no matter how many companies that person had worked for.

Big insurance companies have a lot of money and they intend to keep it. They are also very powerful and many of the lords and MP's who drive our legal system have a vested interest in certain companies as shareholders.

A new ruling is due to be made in **June 2007** which will decide if people suffering from pleural plaques will come under the same banner as those suffering from asbestosis and mesothelioma. At the moment they do not.

Trudy McPhillips had pleural plaques. In 1998 she told me that she had to undertake medical tests to see how ill she was. She was made to walk up stairs and she struggled. The 'experts' decided she wasn't ill enough to receive some benefits *and that pleural plaques did not lead to mesothelioma.*

In 2006 one of the members of Asbestos Action Tayside had pleural plaques. Within weeks he had developed mesothelioma and died. Pleural plaques quite clearly can and do lead to pleural thickening and mesothelioma.

The debate over compensation and what should and should not be termed as a disease caused by asbestos is usually controlled by big powerful and very rich companies who have a vested interest in not being found liable in any way whatsoever. The insurance companies who are made to pay out in compensation cases are also rich and powerful. Money and power talks.

As companies around the globe have denied liability, covered up evidence, suppressed information and lied through their back teeth, making a vast fortune in the process, people who have been exposed to asbestos – and their families – have been dying.

Asbestos is a big, sad word.

It's also an international disaster.

And the whole, sorry tale has, like dust, been swept under the carpet.

BMcK 1995

The Future

The Hidden Plague?

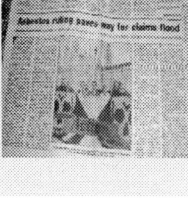

By the time the UK government banned blue asbestos in 1971, it had been firmly established throughout the world (all asbestos was eventually banned in 1999).

By then asbestos fibres were already in the atmosphere and were found in the desert sands of the Middle East and in the air streams of Siberia.

Asbestos is part of our global ecosystem.

Big companies deny anything to do with asbestos. In fact, on 14th November 2005 I overheard a radio program, which said that insurance companies are saying that pleural plaques *should not* be covered or compensated for, because there is not *outward affect* on the victim.

* * * * * *

If you look on the web, take a look at the latest breaking news at

http://www.mesolink.org/mesothelioma-news/

Funeral Takes Place
For 9/11 EMT Worker

The funeral has taken place for an EMT worker who worked at Ground Zero in New York after the 9/11 tragedy, and then went on to develop the asbestos related cancer Mesothelioma, from which she died.

Shopping Centre Delay Due To Asbestos

The development of a shopping centre in Milford has been put on hold due to a problem with naturally occurring asbestos.

Mother Angered Over School Asbestos Removal

A mother from Vancouver has revealed that she may be taking legal action over the removal of asbestos near to her 8-year-old daughter's spring break day care class.

Majority of Indians Against Asbestos Ship

Following the recent controversy surrounding the French ship, the Clemenceau, which was said to contain hundreds of tons of asbestos, it has been revealed that around 70% of Indians are against the vessel being broken up in India.

* * * * * *

Or go to the BBC news website (http://news.bbc.co.uk/) and search on ASBESTOS you will find over 30 pages of articles relating to asbestos. Here are a few…

Asbestos closes Brixton station

Brixton's tube station in south London shuts for nine days while asbestos is removed..

School closes after asbestos find

A school in the south Wales valleys is closed after asbestos is discovered during a site review..

New warning over hidden asbestos

The TUC claim that millions of people could be working in buildings with asbestos.

Firm sprayed asbestos into river

C&W Roofing of Hythe Quay disposed of waste from jet spray washings into the River Lee. Asbestos fibres had worked its way into Luton's sewage system and some of the liquid which was on a grass verge had dried out, causing asbestos fibres to go into the air.

Warning over asbestos fire debris

Debris from a large fire at B&Q at Branston, Burton-On-Trent, which contains asbestos is found in South Derbyshire, Brizlincote Valley and Stapenhill.

Firm fined over factory asbestos

Asbestos was found in production areas of an egg box factory, Omni-Pac at Great Yarmouth. The company fined £136,000 for 'potentially exposing staff to asbestos'

Residents discuss asbestos site

Developers want to build 650 new homes on the site of a former asbestos factory (previously owned by Turner & Newall) in Rochdale. Asbestos had been found on the site and the developers, MMC Estates and Countryside Properties twice failed to disclose this fact. Locals got together to discuss the issue.

Anger over illegal asbestos dump

Several tonnes of asbestos were illegally dumped on a remote lane in a forest at Mullaghbane, near Forkhill, South Armagh.

Crews tackle straw fires at farms

Fire-fighters had to decontaminate the scene of a farm fire in Kent after asbestos was discovered. 2,000 tonnes of straw were destroyed.

Asbestos death ruled accidental

A Barry Welch, a **32 year old** father of three, died of Mesothelioma. He was exposed to asbestos fibres from his step-dads clothes. His step-dad worked as a scaffolder at a power station in Kent in the 1970's.

* * * * * *

Asbestos is everywhere.

It is in schools, factories, towns, and homes.

It is in the Earth's ecosystem.

It finds its way around our planet, carried by wind and by sea.

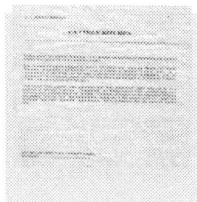

According to the British Journal
of Cancer [19] , deaths from
mesothelioma will peak at
around 2015 (8 years from now).

In 1968 there were 153 reported deaths from
mesothelioma. By 2001 there were 1,848. The
prediction is that in the years 2011 to 2015,
1,950-2,450 people will die of this disease
every year. They say;

> *The eventual death rate will depend on the background
> level and any residual asbestos exposure. Between
> 1968 and 2050, there will have been approximately
> 90 000 deaths from mesothelioma in Great Britain,
> 65 000 of which will occur after 2001.*

However, as has been noted through-out this
book, death certificates do not always state
that asbestos or related diseases were
responsible for the death of someone, which
means that many more people have died than
is actually recorded in any government
statistics.

---

[19] http://www.nature.com/bjc (government statistics)

According to the TUC [20] over **5,000** people a year are currently dying from an asbestos related disease in the UK. That's twice the estimate of official government peak number of the future. Figures, from 1990-2001 show the following [21];

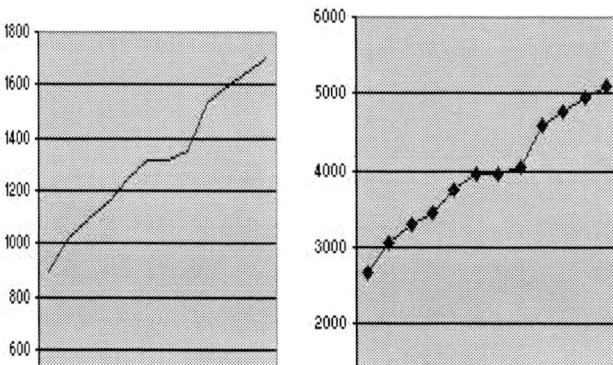

UK Deaths 1990-2001
mesothelioma (left) and all asbestos related (right)

In 1990, 1705 people died of an asbestos related disease. By 2001, the estimated number was 5115, that's a 300% increase within 10 years.

---

[20] Trades Union Congress http://www.tuc.org.uk/

[21] TUC Source: mesothelioma deaths from 1990-1999 are taken from *Health and Safety Statistics 2001* published by the HSE, and are based on death certificates issued in England, Scotland and Wales. * The projected fatalities for 2000 and 2001 are based on the average annual increase from the previous five years – see website for further details

---

The author of the book *Asbestos Killer Dust*, Alan Dalton, spoke on behalf of the TUC Hazards Campaign in 2002. He is quoted here,

> "If the millions of tonnes of asbestos in our homes, schools, hospitals and workplaces is not removed and disposed of safely the 'asbestos cancer epidemic' will continue well into the 22nd century. We must get it right this time, for our children's grandchildren!"

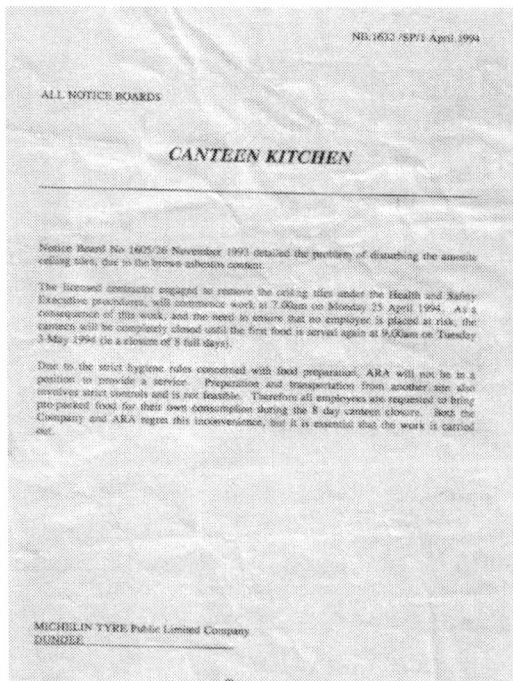

NB. 1632 /SP/1 April 1994

ALL NOTICE BOARDS

CANTEEN KITCHEN

Notice Board No. 1605/26 November 1993 detailed the problem of disturbing the asbestos ceiling tiles, due to the brown asbestos content.

The licensed contractor engaged to remove the ceiling tiles under the Health and Safety Executive procedures, will commence work at 7.00am on Monday 25 April 1994. As a consequence of this work, and the need to ensure that no employee is placed at risk, the canteen will be completely closed until the first food is served again at 9.00am on Tuesday 3 May 1994 (ie a closure of 8 full days).

Due to the strict hygiene rules concerned with food preparation, ARA will not be in a position to provide a service. Preparation and transportation from another site also involves strict controls and is not feasible. Therefore all employees are requested to bring pre-packed food for their own consumption during the 8 day canteen closure. Both the Company and ARA regret this inconvenience, but it is essential that the work is carried out.

MICHELIN TYRE Public Limited Company
DUNDEE

A notice posted by Michelin Tyre, Dundee
for their employees 1994

The World Today

In 1999 the importation, sale and new use of **all** asbestos was banned in the UK and Europe.

The first country in the European Union to ban all forms of asbestos was Sweden in 1982 [22]. Swedish authorities had also brought in measures to control and reduce asbestos importation and use in their country in the mid 1970's.

Due to these actions, Sweden is now the only European country where deaths due to exposure to asbestos, has been declining.

In direct contrast to this, the use of asbestos is rising in India [23] Even although white asbestos mining is banned there, the import, export and manufacturing use of it is permitted. It is currently being used for water, sewage & drainage pipes, packing materials, car brake linings and more.

---

[22] European Asbestos Campaign 2006
http://www.hvbg.de/e/asbest/

[23] see chapter *Mumbai, India*

An article in the India Times (July 2006)[24] states;

> "Studies reveal that the demand for asbestos in India is around 100,000 tonnes, a fifth of which is mined domestically.
>
> In addition, raw asbestos worth Rs.100 million is imported every year mainly from Canada and Russia, the two major producers of the mineral"

In India Subrata Dutta, the communications officer of Mine Labour Protection Campaign (a Jodhpur-based NGO), has stated that studies in India have found a high incidence of asbestos related diseases amongst workers and that those workers are unaware of and uneducated about the dangers.

Even although asbestos mining is banned by the Indian government, Dutta said;

> "But in many mining areas of Rajasthan, asbestos is still extracted and traded"

---

[24] India Times
http://timesofindia.indiatimes.com/articleshow/1758020.cms

Asbestos is a killer.

It does not care what colour your skin is.
It does not care what language you speak.
It does not care how old you are.
It does not care who your Gods are.

It is a very deadly mineral and it kills, very
slowly and very painfully.

Asbestos is a big, sad word.

It's also an international disaster.

And the whole, sorry tale is still, like dust,
being swept under the carpet.

BMcK 2007

Me & Mum

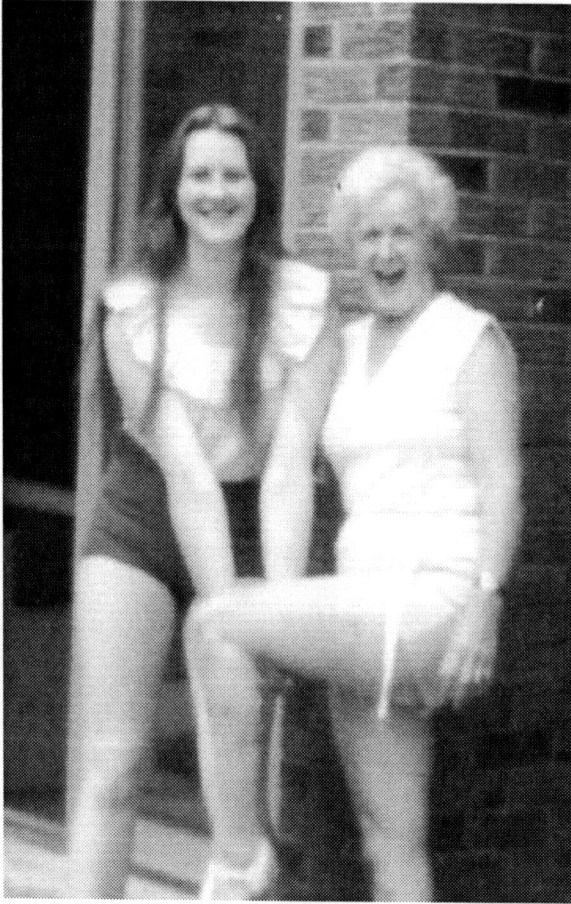

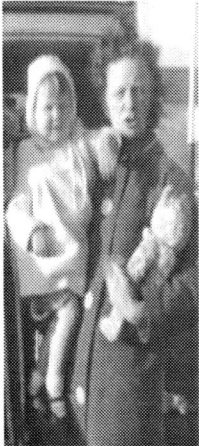
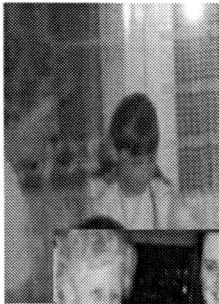
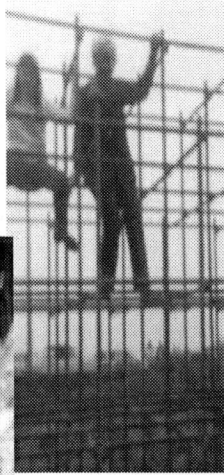
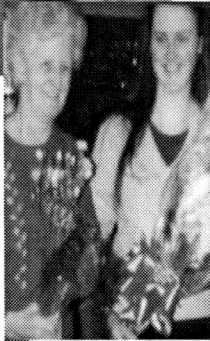
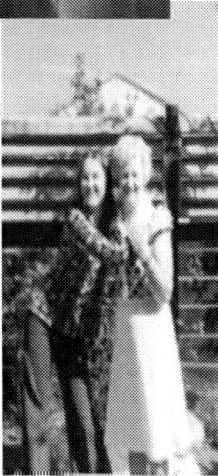
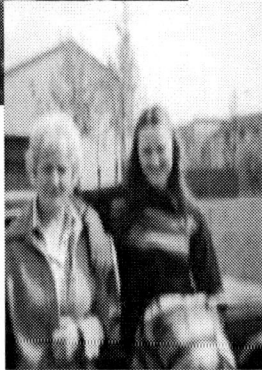
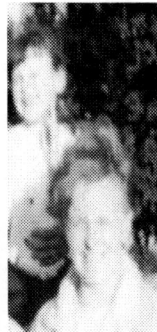

"No-one Knows What I'm Going Through"

Ellen Whitelaw McKessock, 1993

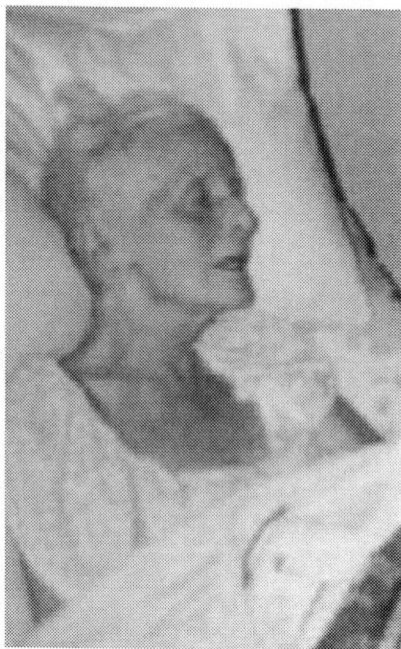

References

Books

Mesothelioma; the story of an illness,
B McKessock (Argyll Publishing 1995) *Out Of Print*

Blue Murder, Ben Hills (Sun Books, Australia 1989)

Asbestos Killer Dust, Alan Dalton ()

Steve McQueen – the untold story of a bad boy in Hollywood, Penina Spiegel
(William Collins, Glasgow, 1986)

Medicines – the comprehensive guide
(Parragon, 1993)

Booklets & Reports

Asbestos Killer Dust (BSSRS Publications Ltd, 1979), **Asbestos – what you should know** (Asbestos Diseases Society of Australia), **Mesothelioma Research Report** (National Cancer Institute), **Victims Twice Over**, Joanne Lenaghan (East End Management Committee, 1994), **Hull Asbestos Action Group** (Reports 1990-93)

Leaflets

Asbestos in Housing (Department of the Environment), **Lung Cancer – the facts**, Chris Williams (Oxford University Press, 1992), **the facts about your lungs – Asbestosis** (British Lung Foundation), **the way our lungs work** (British Lung Foundation), **when someone with cancer is dying** (Cancerlink, 1991), **life with cancer** (Cancerlink), **voluntary euthanasia – your questions answered** (VESS, 1992), **PN1 Pneumoconiosis, byssinosis & some other diseases** (Benefits Agency, 1992)

Online Sources
**Mesothelioma Mortality in Great Britain,
An Analysis by Geographical Area 1981-2000**
Health & Safety Executive – National Statistics
http://www.hse.gov.uk/statistics/causdis/area8100.pdf

British Asbestos Newsletter
http://www.lkaz.demon.co.uk/ban18.htm

Asbestos, Great Britain's Runaway Killer
http://www.hazards.org/haz74/asbestosconcern.pdf

**Asbestosis in an asbestos composite mill at
Mumbai: A prevalence study**
V Murlidhar & Vijay Kanhere
http://www.pubmedcentral.nih.gov/picrender.fcgi?ar
tid=1289287&blobtype=pdf

India Times – asbestos use rising
http://timesofindia.indiatimes.com/articleshow/1758
020.cms

TUC
http://www.tuc.org.uk/the_tuc/tuc-4392-f0.cfm

British Journal of Cancer
http://www.nature.com/bjc/journal/v92/n3/full/66
02307a.html

Chase Manhattan's Unlikely Heroics
http://www.motherjones.com/news/outfront/1993/
11/woody.html

The Current Asbestos Situation in Sweden
http://www.hvbg.de/e/asbest/konfrep/konfrep/rep
beitr/traegardh_en.pdf

Steve McQueen
http://www.stevemcqueen.org.uk/
http://www.mcqueenonline.com/

Mesothelioma http://www.mesolink.org/

BBC news website http://news.bbc.co.uk/

Newspaper Articles & Information from;
Chicago Tribune, Courier & Advertiser, Daily Express,
Daily Mirror, Daily Record, Evening Courier, Evening
Times, Glasgow Herald, The Guardian, Halifax Courier,
Hebden Bridge Times, Hull Daily Mail, Mail On Sunday,
Northern Star, Sunday Express, Sunday Mail,
Sunday Post, The Times, Yorkshire Post

Other Sources
Private Diaries : Ellen Whitelaw McKessock (1992) & B
McKessock (1992/93), Photographs : McKessock Family

Links

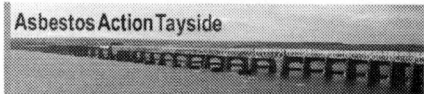

Asbestos Action Tayside
C/o Digby Brown, Royal Exchange,
Panmure Street, Dundee DD1 1DU
http://www.asbestosactiontayside.org.uk

Clydeside Action on Asbestos
245 High Street, Glasgow, G4 0QR
Tel: 0141 552 8852

June Hancock Mesothelioma Research Fund
http://www.leeds.ac.uk/meso/index.htm

British Asbestos Newsletter
http://www.lkaz.demon.co.uk

International Ban Asbestos Secretariat
http://www.ibas.btinternet.co.uk/

Mesothelioma UK
http://www.mesothelioma.uk.com/

Trades Union Congress (TUC)
A series of TUC rights leaflets are available on our
website and from the
know your rights line 0870 600 4 882
Lines are open every day from 8am-10pm
Calls are charged at the national rate
http://www.tuc.org.uk/